Periods...Just Why?

A No-Nonsense Guide to Mastering your Hormones and Menstrual Cycle.

Bernice Pond

PERIODS…JUST WHY?

TABLE OF CONTENTS

ABOUT THE AUTHOR

My name is Bernice Pond SRN (State Registered Nurse), and I'm a happily retired nurse. For 40 years, I had an extensive, eventful and fulfilling career. During my time in the nursing profession, I was able to work with people from all countries and walks of life. I have seen and heard pretty much everything you can think of, little shocks me those days.

Now that I have retired, I have been able to turn my attention towards three neglected passions of mine - reading books, writing books and trying to bake lovely cakes and biscuits! I'm currently enjoying the comforts of a writing desk and an unlimited supply of coffee and biscuits. I share my home with one busy daughter, one grumpy husband and two demanding cats.

INTRODUCTION

Let me tell you a story about a young, 11-year-old girl.

One day while at school, she went to use the bathroom, but she found something strange on her underwear: blood. That was not something she normally saw when she went to the bathroom. She had no clue what was going on and was too afraid to ask her mother or friends about it.

She suddenly remembered seeing something in biology class about this. She thought to herself, "This must be the **period** they were talking about!"

She folded up some toilet paper in a frantic hurry and placed it in her underwear. The only thing she could think to do was sneak to the store later that day, to try and buy something for the blood. She remembered the teacher talking about pads and tampons for this sort of thing.

Standing there in the aisle, staring at all the different varieties, she had no clue what she needed. Tears started to well up in her eyes. She decided to grab a package with some pretty flowers on it, and then she walked up to the cashier while desperately trying to avoid eye contact. She quickly paid for her pads and rushed home, staring at the ground the entire way.

When the little girl returns home, the only guidance she will have are the directions on the package. Beyond that, no one will be there to tell her what to do about this incident. Situations like this happen every day. What this girl didn't realise then was that she had just crossed a significant puberty milestone on her way to becoming a woman.

I'm sure you can remember exactly how it *happened* — the first time you got your period. It's just one of those flashbulb memories that you will never forget. It is likely scarred in your mind forever. It was the day you crossed that invisible line between being a young, innocent girl and turning into a mature woman, whose body had started to prime for baby-making.

As women and girls, we all share one common thread: we all have our period!

Having your period is messy. It makes you sore (like being hit by a train); is emotionally draining; is irritating; and not to mention, it's highly inconvenient!

Sadly, there are still many myths and so much confusion surrounding the most natural — and dare I say — *beautiful* parts of a woman's life. While many women view their periods as a curse, what they don't realise is precisely why this monthly annoyance happens. It may be irritating, but there are a lot of processes occurring in your body that makes this phenomenon essential for your reproductive health.

After I had my daughter, I vowed to be different. I wanted to make sure she was educated in the ways of the female body and was never ashamed or embarrassed by this entirely natural process. However, I was astonished by the lack of available resources and practical guides out there for young women, mature women, daughters, and mothers alike. There was nothing that demystified the physical and psychological aspects of why we get periods or hormones and the roles they play during the menstruation cycle. This is the main reason that I was driven to write the book.

For you.

For your daughter.

For your mother.

For your girlfriend.

For your partner.

For anyone with female reproductive organs.

And the men! Guys, you should read this book; you

have a lot to learn too!

It is my goal with this book to be able to answer the most common and pressing questions that you may have, many of the questions courtesy of my daughter. Most of the questions she asked were questions I wondered about myself - before I received my nursing education.

This book contains everything about menstrual health that I wish my mother, or my girlfriends would have told me. I also wrote this book, so I could pass it down to my daughter, and then to her daughter, and future generations after that. I hope that mothers and daughters can share the journey of womanhood with knowledge and confidence in the future.

I also want to dispel any key myths that continue to linger around the subject of periods and the menstrual cycle. We all know that knowledge is power, and the knowledge from this book will help make the mysterious world of menstrual cycles more comprehensible. This book will also be a valuable tool for helping you monitor your physical health and well-being.

But first, let me introduce myself.

My name is Bernice Pond, SRN (State Registered Nurse). For forty years, I have had an eventful and fulfilling career as a registered nurse in the UK. I was able to work with many young ladies and women during my years in the nursing profession. People always asked me questions about everything related to periods and menstruation. I have taken the journey from menstruation to menopause while witnessing my friends and colleagues experience the same. During the forty or so years I had my periods, they were always extremely heavy and accompanied by painful PMS symptoms.

I can understand the humiliation of feeling a wet liquid ooze out onto your uniform (this was startling to me when I got my period early). I was also amazed by the side effects that birth control had on my body, such as black blood, thinning hair, and irregular bleeding when coming off the pill.

It is vital to educate yourself and learn the properties of the menstrual cycle. Having this knowledge will teach you how to regulate your menstrual cycle and heighten your awareness of the relationship between your hormones and your body. After reading this book, you will be able to separate period myths from period truths and resolve tough questions about menstruation. This crucial knowledge will allow you to work with your body and your emotions, to effectively navigate your way through your monthly cycle with confidence. Furthermore, you will learn where to turn for further support from doctors, when necessary.

During my forty-year career as a nurse; I assisted many young women and children. I was able to provide practical information and support for the confusing changes their bodies were experiencing during womanhood. In this book, I am going to break down my familiarity and expertise to help you better understand your female reproductive system.

I hope this guide will inspire you with confidence and answer any questions you may be asking yourself about your period.

You could go on guessing, in agony each month when you have your period — having no clue as to why you experience these pains and symptoms. You could try to talk to your friends about the issues you have, but they are likely just as clueless as you are. You could continue believing these silly myths that keep you from enjoying life while on your period.

OR!

You could continue to read this book and arm yourself with the knowledge you need to tackle your menstrual cycle every month confidently.

I have packed every chapter of this book with actionable steps that will help answer all your burning questions and provide you with the assurance you need. You don't need to suffer in silence or scour the internet in search of unreliable or even potentially dangerous answers to your questions! I am going to cover everything every woman should know about periods but have always been too afraid to ask.

Some topics addressed in this book will include:

- Female reproductive biology.
- Myths surrounding periods.
- The purpose of ovulation and menstruation.
- The menstrual cycle step by step and how to track it.
- The physical and psychological effects of your period.
- Birth control and hormonal effects on your period.
- Understanding heavy and painful periods.
- Menstrual care products.
- Lifestyle changes you can make to feel a little better during your period.

And so much more!

So, if you have female reproductive organs (or know someone who does) and would like to have light shed on this complex topic, this book is for you.

I'm not going to bore you with statistics and medical jargon that you aren't going to understand. I've written this book to be enjoyable to read alone, or for teens and adults to read together. I will also be sprinkling some fun facts into the mix, for example:

Fun Fact: Did you know that the average woman has 400 periods in total? That would be about four to six years straight of bleeding in our lifetime.

It doesn't matter if you are just starting to get your period or have gone through the menopause. I can guarantee that you will learn something new, that will help to contribute to your overall health and well-being.

So, let's get down to business!

PERIODS...JUST WHY?

CHAPTER ONE – PERIOD MYTH BUSTER SPECIAL

As with many topics, urban legends and myths plague the issue of menstruation. Everyone has a story of some kind: a home remedy, or superstition about periods and menstruation.

We must recognize that many of these stories are unfounded by science or have been proven entirely false.

For centuries, periods have been stigmatized and misunderstood not only by women but by society as a whole. It's not clear why menstruation was stigmatized. Sigmund Freud said it was because humans feared blood. Some said it was "pollution," or toxic. Many historians blame the stigma on ancient patriarchal societies (or, society lead by men) misunderstanding the female body, usually for lack of formal study of female biology (Druet, 2017).

In this chapter, we will go over some of the common cultural myths surrounding periods. We will also dispel the key urban legends I'm sure you've heard once or twice yourself. Some of them are quite amusing, while others are a little more complicated and may sound like they *could* be the truth.

Periods are a normal part of the female reproductive process, and you should not feel ashamed about them, nor should you have to hide from them.

Cultural Myths

Every culture has its myths and superstitions about various topics. Almost every country has some silly cultural tale about women being on their "time of the month." While most of these myths are utterly foolish, some of them can negatively affect a woman's education, job, safety, and overall equality in many countries (Werft & Canal, 2017).

Cultural Myths Surrounding Food

One of the most significant cultural superstitions that I have seen, again and again, is that women on their period will contaminate the food they are cooking. This belief is found in countries like Italy, India, Japan, France (*any mayonnaise you make will spoil*), Argentina, and even in the US and the UK. The myth is mostly due to menstruating women being regarded as unclean (Werft & Canal, 2017).

One typical food-related myth in the US and UK is that if you touch vegetables meant for pickling while on your period, they will not ferment properly and spoil as a result (Clue, 2017).

Cultural Myths Surrounding Cleanliness

There are numerous cultural myths surrounding menstruation and cleanliness.

Some people in the US and UK believe that you shouldn't perm your hair until after you have had your first period. This opinion may have more to do with the chemicals used in the perming process and less to do with actual menstruation.

Several countries believe that you shouldn't take a bath or shower while menstruating. Israelis believe that if you shower with hot water, your flow will be much heavier.

No thanks, I will take my nice warm showers!

Many cultures believe that if you shower or bathe while menstruating, you can become infertile, or cause others you are living with to become sick. This idea is not true — you should bathe or shower while on your period! Showering and bathing have no ill effect on your fertility or menstruation. If you don't shower and bathe, not only are you going to smell of body odour, there is an increased chance of infection. Moreover, taking a bath or shower can help stop your period during that time (Clue, 2017).

They believe, in Colombia, that you should not wash or cut your hair while on your period (Clue, 2017). In India, they think that if you shower or wash your hair, your flow will decrease, thus decreasing your chances of fertility.

In places like India, Bali, and Nepal, women are not allowed to enter places of worship, and this idea can circle back to cleanliness. Temples are considered clean and holy places; when women are menstruating, they are deemed "unclean." It is a terrible example of gender inequality around the world (Werft & Canal, 2017).

In Nepal, if you are a woman who is experiencing menstruation, you are unable to enter homes or be in contact with other people. In an ancient Hindu practice called *chhaupadi*, Nepalese women are forced to live in *special huts* while they are experiencing menstruation. These huts are usually dirty and have terrible living conditions (Cousins, 2019). *Chhaupadi* is also a common practice in parts of India and Bangladesh. They believe that period blood is impure. This treatment sends a signal to women and young girls that they are dirty and inferior to their male counterparts (Cousins, 2019). It's an archaic practice that has even led to death as women are exposed to extreme elements while living in mud and straw huts for the time of their menstruation.

Chhaupadi also effectively hinders women from attending worship, work, or school. The myths surrounding menstruation as unclean is causing a huge economic problem in many countries, merely because of a lack of education.

Cultural Myths Surrounding Animals

Yes, you read that right. There are myths about menstruation surrounding *animals*.

Some people in the US believe that you should avoid going camping while on your period as bears will be able to smell the blood and will attack you (Clue, 2017).

Sharks are another animal that can apparently smell period blood. According to some people, sharks will strike at a menstruating woman if she is in the water. This is despite there being no data to back up that claim. So, you shouldn't be too quick to blame periods for indiscriminate shark attacks (Werft & Canal, 2017).

Fun Fact: While all mammals go through gestation and birth babies (rather than hatching them), only primates, elephants, shrews, and bats experience a monthly menstrual cycle as humans do.

Other Silly Cultural Myths

Some people in the US and UK believe that you are clumsier on your period. While menstruation is not a common cause of clumsiness, pregnancy can make you clumsier. As you progress in pregnancy, your centre of gravity is thrown off, making it more likely that you will trip over your own feet.

This myth is one I'm sure you've heard at least once in your life, and it goes something like this. If you wear a tampon before losing your virginity, it will break your hymen. As a result, you will become "impure." The truth is, whether your hymen is intact has nothing to do with your virginity. The hymen is merely a small membrane just inside the opening of the vagina. While historically it was used to determine a woman's virginity, it can be worn away or broken by activities other than sexual intercourse. Other activities that can break the hymen include horseback riding, gymnastics, or the use of a tampon. Not all women have the same kind of hymen. It is like a piece of tissue paper and can be broken or torn easily (Wischhover, 2019; Tanner & Briganti, 2015). The idea of a hymen and virginity is meant to control women and deter them from having sex (Tanner & Briganti, 2015).

We have all heard the jokes about premenstrual syndrome, or PMS, and how it manifests into crankiness and irritability. While yes, some women may experience PMS, not all women experience the crankiness and irritability. Many women experience other symptoms like bloating, fatigue, and acne. For a long time, PMS has been synonymous with "that time of the month," but it shouldn't be. Experiencing PMS and all its symptoms is a natural and healthy part of being a woman (National Health Service [NHS], 2018).

Here are some fun ones…

In Poland, they believe that having sex with your partner while menstruating will kill them (Clue, 2017). Not sure what the actual reasoning is behind this one, but I guess it's a bit of an excuse to avoid sex while on your period if you're not in the mood.

In Mexico, you should protect your uterus by avoiding dancing to very active and rhythmic beats (Clue, 2017).

In Venezuela, your skin will get darker if you shave your bikini line while on your period (Clue, 2017).

In the Philippines, you should take the blood from

your first period and wash your face with it to have clear skin. How lovely. This one kind of sounds like some weird ritual out of a horror movie (Clue, 2017).

In Brazil, they believe that if you walk barefoot while menstruating, you will get cramps (Clue, 2017).

In Bolivia, you are not supposed to cradle a baby while on your period, or you will cause them to get sick (Clue, 2017). There's something a little odd about this one. What about after you give birth and are bleeding? Are you not supposed to hold your baby? You can see how silly some of these myths are. Most of them stemmed from some Old Wives tales that some cultures cannot seem to let go.

So, to recap, some of the most basic cultural myths include not exposing yourself to water, not touching any food or plants, and staying away from predatory animals and other people in general. Therefore, according to these myths, all menstruating women should be quarantined.

I don't think so!

Of course, there are those urban legends that float around online and in teen groups that don't always have obvious answers. You may have heard some myths from your friends or your mother or grandmother. Many of them are not accurate, and they're just tales that have been passed from generation to generation until they are believed indefinitely by the next generation.

So, we're going to go ahead and bust ten common urban legends that exist in the US and the UK.

1. You Can't Get Pregnant During Your Period

I've heard this one a lot during my time as a nurse. What many women believe is that when you are on your period, you are shedding your lining; therefore, an egg cannot become fertilized. This assumption is INCORRECT. What many women don't realize is that sperm can live in the uterine lining for up to five days with ovulation occurring before, during, or after the bleeding phase (Miller, 2019).

You are indeed less fertile during the actual menstruation phase of your monthly cycle. Be careful if you are having unprotected sex during your period.

Sperm can stick around long enough to come in contact with an egg and fertilize it (Cohut, 2019). This occurrence does result in pregnancy.

Furthermore, if you have unprotected sex on your period, you are at a higher risk of contracting sexually transmitted infections (STIs) or a yeast infection. You are at a higher risk during this time due to the increase in certain hormones (Cohut, 2019).

You absolutely can get pregnant if you have sex on your period, so you should plan accordingly.

2. Irregular Periods are Bad for Your Reproductive Health

Many women experience irregular periods. If you think you have missed a period, you should consult with your doctor or take a pregnancy test (if you are sexually active). When you first get your period, it can take anywhere from six to twelve months to "become regular" (Miller, 2019)

Some women never experience a regular period, and that too is entirely normal. Many things can contribute to the onset of irregular periods, such as stress, diet, exercise, and illness (Miller, 2019). Again, it's always a good idea to talk to your doctor if you're concerned.

3. Menstrual Cycles are Only Twenty-Eight Days Long

As with the previous myth, many women have irregular periods. The twenty-eight day cycle is only an estimate and an average for lots of women. If you are having trouble determining your period cycle, try tracking it to get a better idea as to when you will get your period. Calendars, charts, and phone apps are great ways to track your period schedule.

4. Menstrual Blood is Different than Regular Blood

This one is a little upsetting to think about, especially after having just discussed cultural myths. When it comes to your body, blood is blood, whether it comes out of your nose or your vagina. Menstrual blood is thought of often as different blood because it comes out of the vagina for several days at a time. If any other part of you were bleeding this long, you would likely pass out from loss of blood. Menstrual blood can also look different because it's mixed with mucus and other vaginal discharge.

5. Bed Rest is a Must During Your Period

While this myth can be a great excuse to get out of housework and other responsibilities, bed rest is not necessary. You should try to be active during your period just like you would any other day of the month. While cramping can leave you feeling bedridden, light exercise can help to relieve some of that cramping (Miller, 2019). It also helps to release endorphins and other feel-good hormones, helping to lift your mood.

6. You Can't Have Sex During Your Period

Nothing is stopping you from having sex on your period, except you (or your partner).

Many women choose to wait due to the potential mess, menstrual cramping or based on religious beliefs (Gallagher, 2017). There is nothing to be ashamed about when it comes to having sex on your period. It is completely natural. If your partner is uncomfortable with it, talk to them and educate them on why it isn't unclean.

Although I would suggest, you grab an extra towel so, you don't get your sheets dirty.

7. Your Period Can Become Synchronized With Other Ladies

Anyone who has lived with multiple women (roommates, family members, etc.) likely knows what *Shark Week* is. It is a term given when multiple women live together and sync up their periods. While many believe that period syncing is a real phenomenon, the research study that claimed such in the '70s turned out to be unreliable because the findings were never able to be replicated. The researcher's methodology was also questionable (Cohut, 2019). Therefore, any synching up of periods is simply a coincidence.

8. You Shouldn't Take a Bath During Your Period

The myth of not bathing or showering stems from the belief that hot water can cause more bleeding or that the water can stop the bleeding, creating additional ill effects (Cohut, 2019). It has more to do with physics than anything else. When you fully submerge yourself in water, the pressure of the water stops blood from flowing out of the vagina (Cohut, 2019). There are no ill effects to having a bath or shower while menstruating. It is an excellent way for you to relax a bit. A warm bath can help to relieve cramps and help to ease other symptoms of menstruation.

When choosing personal hygiene products, it is better to go mild. Warm water, unscented soaps, and wipes are the best options for cleaning during your period. Many products can disrupt the delicate Ph balance of your vagina and cause infection (Cohut, 2019). You should also try to avoid getting soap inside the vagina; it is like a self-cleaning oven, so you only need to wipe down the outside.

9. You Can't Exercise or Go Swimming During Your Period

You might want to take it a little easier during your period. However, if you experience severe PMS symptoms, there is no reason to stop exercising or go swimming during your period. Doing most of your regular exercise will benefit you. Cardio and light strength training can help to ease cramps and improve your overall well-being (Bodyform, 2016).

Physical activity also helps to relieve stress, releasing the hormones dopamine and serotonin. Dopamine is the "happy" hormone that helps to decrease stress and elevate your mood. The release of serotonin helps you to get a good night's rest while improving mood and sexual function (Piedmont Healthcare [PH], 2019).

10. You Can Pass Out from Period Blood Loss

While it might look like you are losing a lot of blood while you are menstruating, it's not as much as you think. You are generally only losing between two to three tablespoons of blood during each menstruation (Bodyform, 2016). Some women may experience more blood loss than others due to heavier periods, but you shouldn't be feeling weak or dizzy. If you are, you should speak with your doctor about your symptoms.

So, the next time someone says something silly about how you shouldn't take a bath or cook particular foods while on your period, educate them! Even better, suggest they read this book.

There is nothing wrong or shameful about having your period. It's a perfectly natural and beautiful thing that only women get to experience.

Chapter Summary

There are many cultural myths and urban legends surrounding menstruation; most of them are pretty silly, whereas others jeopardize women's safety. Myths and cultural stigmas surrounding periods perpetuate gender inequality in many countries. Here is a list of myths and misbeliefs that people from all over the world believe in:

- Menstruating women will contaminate any food or person they touch.
- Menstruating women are unclean.
- Menstruating women can't bathe or shower.
- Touching food that is meant to ferment will spoil it.
- You shouldn't perm your hair before your first period.

- Showering or bathing can make a person infertile or make others around you sick.
- Showering with hot water causes your flow to become heavier.
- You shouldn't wash or cut your hair while menstruating.
- Bears will smell your blood and attack you if you camp while menstruating.
- Sharks will smell your menstrual blood and attack you.
- You are clumsier on your period.
- Using tampons will break your hymen and take your virginity.
- All women become irritated during their time of the month.
- Having sex on your period will kill your partner.
- Dancing to very active and rhythmic beats can damage your uterus.
- Shaving your bikini line while menstruating will cause your skin to become darker.
- Walking barefoot will cause cramping.
- Holding a baby while menstruating will cause them to get sick.

- You can't get pregnant during your period.

- Irregular periods are bad for your reproductive health.

- Menstrual cycles always last exactly twenty-eight days.

- Menstrual blood isn't regular blood.

- You must be on strict bed rest while on your period.

- Your period will sync with other ladies whom you spend a lot of time.

- You can't exercise or swim during your period.

- You can pass out from period blood loss.

As you can see, there are many silly myths out there.

In the next chapter, we are going to discuss the biology behind why you have periods in the first place. We also delve into everything you ever wanted (or didn't want to know) about the female reproductive system.

CHAPTER TWO – BIOLOGY 101 – WHY DO YOU HAVE PERIODS IN THE FIRST PLACE?

Now we have covered the common and not so common myths surrounding periods. So, let's dive into the biology behind the menstruation cycle.

In this chapter, I am going to outline the female reproductive system, how it works and what happens during puberty. I will also cover the typical age someone will experience their first period, and the length of time a woman will experience her periods.

The Female Reproductive System

The female reproductive system is a fantastic part of every woman's body. It serves several purposes and can carry out several functions (Johnson, 2018). The reproductive system produces the egg necessary for fertilization. If the egg becomes fertilized, it results in a pregnancy. However, if the egg does not become fertilized, then menstruation takes place, and the inner lining of the uterine wall will shed. Lastly, the female reproductive system is responsible for maintaining the reproductive cycle through the production of female sex hormones (Johnson, 2019).

Female reproductive organs serve four main purposes (Hirsch, 2019):

- To produce eggs.
- To have sexual intercourse.
- To protect and nourish a fertilized egg through gestation.
- To give birth.

There are two main sections of the female reproductive system: the *internal* and the *external*, or the **genitalia**. Let's first start with the outside of the reproductive system, the **vulva**.

Mons Pubis

Otherwise known as *pubic hair*. Detection of these hairs in the armpits and pubic area is one of the onset signs of puberty for young girls. The mons pubis is explicitly the fatty area surrounding the pelvic bone that grows hair during puberty.

Clitoris

The clitoris is the only organ that is meant entirely for pleasure. It is like the head of the male penis and covered by a fold of skin. Much like a penis, the clitoris is very sensitive to stimulation and can also become erect when stimulated (Johnson, 2019).

Labia Majora

The outermost part of the vagina. It acts as a protective barrier to the internal sexual organs. The labia majora are also referred to as the "large lips" of the vagina. They will become covered in hair after the onset of puberty. Like other areas of the skin, they can sweat and secrete oil (Johnson, 2019).

Labia Minora

The labia minora lay just inside the labia majora and are referred to as the "small lips." They surround the opening of the vagina and urethra (Johnson, 2019). The two sections of the labia minora connect at the top to cover the clitoris and form what is called a clitoral hood.

Urethral Opening

The urethral opening is where the bladder connects to the outside of the body. This area is where urine passes out of the body.

Vagina

The vagina is the canal that links the cervix *(see cervix)* to the outside of the body. The vagina can be found on both the inside and outside of the body. This area is where sexual intercourse happens and where babies come out.

Anus

The outermost part of the colon in which waste is passed out of the body.

Anatomy of Vulva

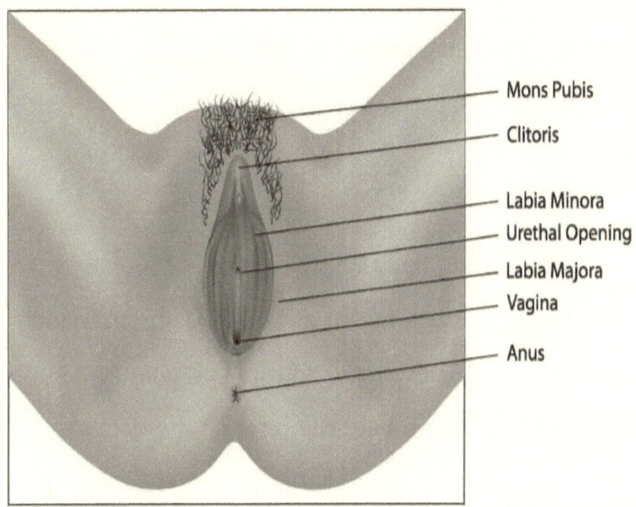

The second part of the female reproductive system is the internal components and is where menstruation, ovulation, and pregnancy all take place.

Vagina

The vagina is both internal and external. What you see in the image below is the inner part of the vagina. As you can see, it's what connects the internal reproductive organs to the external part of the body. The vagina then leads to the cervix. The vagina serves three primary purposes (Hirsch, 2019):

- Sexual intercourse.
- The birth canal.
- Where menstrual blood exits.

Cervix

The cervix is the lower part of the uterus, also known as the neck of the uterus. It is about an inch long with a cylindrical shape. During pregnancy, the cervix dilates to accommodate the birth of the baby.

Uterus

The uterus is a pear-shaped organ that remains hollow unless a fetus is developing. The larger part of the uterus expands to hold the developing baby. The cervix is also what allows sperm to enter the reproductive system, and where menstrual blood passes out of the body.

Fallopian Tubes

The fallopian tubes connect the ovaries to the

uterus. Eggs travel through the fallopian tubes where fertilization takes place. Once an egg moves from the ovary to the fallopian tube and is fertilized, it moves to the uterus where it will then be implanted into the uterine wall for gestation.

Ovaries

The Ovaries are where the eggs are stored. The ovaries are small, egg-shaped glands that sit on either side of the uterus, connected via the fallopian tubes. Not only do the ovaries produce eggs, but they also produce hormones. Ovaries are also called gonads (*nope, this term is not just used for testicles!*).

Fun Fact: A woman is born with all the eggs she will ever produce in a lifetime. This means that when your grandmother was pregnant with your mother, she was also carrying you via your mother's eggs!

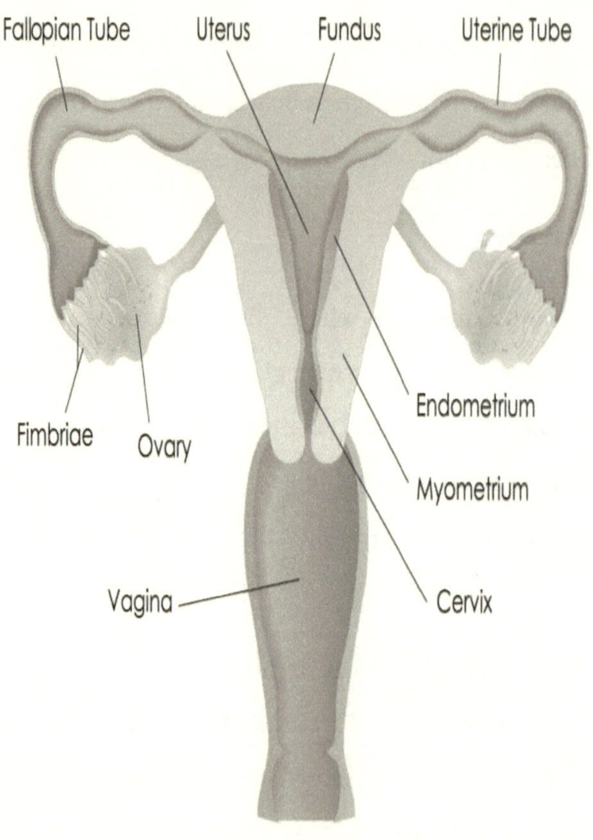

Fallopian Tube
Uterus
Fundus
Uterine Tube
Fimbriae
Ovary
Endometrium
Myometrium
Vagina
Cervix

During Puberty

People experience puberty as a gateway to adulthood. During puberty, a girl's body starts to develop more shape and distributes fat to different areas of the body. Other than infancy, your body grows faster during puberty than any other time in your life (Dowshen, 2015). Puberty is something that everyone experiences. Although everyone experiences puberty a little differently, there are certainly some commonalities that all girls experience.

Below are some of the changes girls go through during puberty.

Hormonal Changes

Puberty starts with the onset of gonadotropin-releasing hormone (or GnRH for short) discharging from the brain (Dowshen, 2015). Puberty generally begins between the ages of seven and thirteen but is highly dependent on many factors. Once GnRH is released, it travels to the pituitary gland. This triggers the release of two more puberty hormones; luteinizing hormone (LH) and follicle-stimulating hormone (FSH; Dowshen, 2015).

Both girls and boys experience this release of the hormone; however, a person's sex affects how the hormones will behave with different parts of the body. In girls, LH and FSH affect the eggs in the ovaries, which have been inactive there since birth.

Girls also experience a growth spurt over the next two to three years during puberty while they transition from being a girl to a woman. It's common for girls to grow up to about four inches per year (Dowshen, 2015). After puberty has ended, you will be your full adult height.

Weight gain is another side effect of puberty. Fat is gained and distributed into the curvier parts of the body: the breasts, hips, and thighs. When girls start to develop breasts, it is common for one to grow unevenly, but they will even out as they further develop.

It can be extremely unhealthy for girls to try and stop this weight gain by dieting or excessive exercise. If girls feel they are gaining too much weight, they should consult their doctor as there might be other issues at play other than just puberty.

The first menstrual period, called **menarche**, usually happens somewhere between two and two and a half years after a girl starts to develop (Brennan, 2019). There are thousands of eggs within a girl's two ovaries. At the onset of menstruation, an egg is released from the ovary; if it's not fertilized, it's then released in what we know as a **period**. This period consists of extra blood and uterine tissues that have been building up during the cycle. While the menstrual cycle usually lasts about twenty-eight days, the period only lasts for about five to seven days.

Physical Changes

Many other changes occur in the female body at the onset of puberty. Girls will start to grow hair in their armpits, their genitals, darker hair begins to develop on their arms and legs, and sometimes even on their face. Acne is also a common side effect of puberty as puberty hormones often trigger it. Acne commonly develops on the face, upper back, and upper chest. Puberty hormones also cause body odour. Bad body odour can easily be avoided with proper hygiene and deodorant (Dowshen, 2015).

Mental Changes

With physical changes also comes mental and emotional changes. During puberty, girls tend to experience strong emotions and confusion (Dowshen, 2015). Girls might experience anxiety as their physical appearance changes, and they can quickly become upset and sensitive over things that wouldn't usually bother them.

Being able to talk to someone about these new feelings can be very beneficial. Whether it's an older sibling, a trusted family friend, or even a professional, there is no need to feel ashamed about physical or emotional changes during puberty. Teens will also start to feel a lot of new feelings and emotions when it comes to sex. It's important that young people have a friendly face to talk about their thoughts and emotions during this time.

Late Onset of Periods

While everyone develops at a different rate, it is common for girls not to get their period until they are around fourteen, and in some cases even older. Your body will naturally go through this process by the age of eighteen (NHS, 2019). In some cases, a doctor may recommend blood tests for older girls who haven't experienced the onset of their periods. They will be this to determine hormone levels. Many reasons could cause girls to experience the late onset of a period:

- Genetics (if your mother or sister started menstruating later in life).
- Underweight.
- Hormonal imbalances.
- Athletic (common for dancers and gymnasts).
- Eating disorders.
- Excessive stress or exercise.
- Problems with the ovaries, womb, or vagina.
- Pregnancy (yes, you can get pregnant before your first period, as the ovaries start to release eggs a few months before the onset of menstruation).

If you don't get your period due to hormonal imbalances, a medical professional may recommend hormone therapy. Depending on the cause of the late onset of a period, there are many options for treatment. There are treatments for eating disorders, excessive exercise, and stress.

How Long Will Periods Last in a Lifetime?

As we covered earlier, girls can start menstruating between the ages of seven and thirteen and won't stop until they experience menopause at around age forty-five to fifty-five. So, for about thirty-five to forty years, a woman will experience menstruation.

At the time of birth, a girl will have anywhere between one to two million eggs in her ovaries, with only about 300,000 remaining by the time she hits puberty. Of all these eggs, she will only release about 500 through menstruation (give or take the number of pregnancies she has), which means 400 to 500 periods in a lifetime (OBOS Anatomy & Menstruation Contributors [OBOSAM], 2014)

That's a lot of tampons!

It doesn't sound like a whole lot of fun. Your best bet is to try and find comfort during this long time, as hard as it may seem.

Chapter Summary

Oh, the mysterious vagina. It's crazy how little women know about their lady parts and what each section of the female sexual organs serves. The purpose of the sexual organs is to produce eggs, engage in sexual intercourse, protect and nourish a fertilized egg (fetus), and to give birth.

In short, our bodies have been designed to create and carry a baby.

The vulva is the outermost section of the female reproductive organs and consist of the mons pubis, clitoris, labia majora, labia minora, urethral opening, vagina, and anus. The inner part of the female reproductive system consists of the vagina, cervix, uterus, fallopian tubes, and ovaries. The internal components of the reproductive system are responsible for menstruation, ovulation, and pregnancy.

The vagina serves three primary purposes: for sexual intercourse, as the birth canal, and where menstrual blood exits.

Puberty is the second time in your life where you grow and change rapidly, other than when you were an infant. During puberty, a girl's body changes as fats are distributed into different areas of the body and hormones run rampant. It can be around two years before girls get their period after puberty has officially started.

Some of the changes that girls experience at the onset of puberty, other than menstruating are:

- Fat distributing to curvier parts of the body.
- Hair growth on the genitals, armpits, and legs.
- Acne or other skin issues.
- Bad body odour.
- Strong emotions.
- Confusion.
- Anxiety.
- Feelings about sex.

Most girls will start to get their periods between the ages of eight to thirteen. However, some girls might experience the late onset of their period. The delayed onset of a period may be due to genetics, weight, athleticism, stress, diet, or reproductive issues.

Women menstruate for about forty years, give or take.

In the next chapter, we are going to decode the menstrual cycle and learn about what hormones do.

CHAPTER THREE – THE MENSTRUAL CYCLE DECODED – WHY HORMONES DO WHAT THEY DO BEST

Many women think that their menstrual cycle only lasts a few days and is just inconvenient and uncomfortable bleeding.

But did you know that your cycle lasts *a lot longer than that?*

The menstrual cycle comprises of four different stages.

In this chapter, we will outline the four stages of your menstrual cycle and how your hormones can affect your menstrual cycle. Finally, we will delve into everything you could ever want to know (or not know) about vaginal discharge.

Why Do You Even Have a Menstrual Cycle?

Every girl and woman is unique. While many women experience menstrual cycles that last five to seven days, others can experience ones that are much shorter or much longer. Several different factors can influence how long a woman's menstrual cycle will last (Liu, Gold, Lasley, & Johnson, 2004):

- Alcohol consumption.
- Smoking.
- Drug use.
- Ethnicity.
- Physical activity level.
- Bodyweight.
- Caffeine consumption.
- Age.
- Medical conditions.

Periods that are longer and irregular seem to normalize with age and rises with an increase in body mass index (Rowland et al., 2002). In a study conducted in 2002, women with a BMI of 35 or higher were twice as likely to have a longer cycle compared to women with a lower BMI. Women who experienced menarche before the age of twelve were more likely to endure shorter and lighter periods. However, if menarche occurred at age fifteen or older, women were more likely to experience heavier period symptoms. Smoking also correlated to drastically shortened and irregular menstrual cycles (Rowland et al.).

How Hormones Affect the Menstrual Cycle

As we discussed earlier, puberty starts due to the release of specific hormones into your body and brain. These hormones serve different functions throughout each stage of menstruation.

During the **follicular phase**, the volume of the hormone **estrogen** increases and the levels of **progesterone** (another type of hormone) lower. This stage is where you are going to feel your best, with more pleasing skin and lots of energy (Klepchukova, 2019). Estrogen plays a massive role in women's health, including but not limited to bone health, mood stability, cholesterol levels, and appearance of skin.

When your estrogen levels reach their peak as a result of positive feedback, luteinizing (LH) levels also increase. Once this happens, **ovulation** takes place.

After ovulation is over and LH and estrogen levels drop, the **luteal phase** begins. During this phase, your body is preparing for pregnancy and progesterone levels increase. Progesterone is "pro-gestational," meaning that it helps support implantation and pregnancy. At this time during the cycle, many women experience PMS symptoms. PMS often manifests as an increase in appetite, fatigue, skin issues, and oily skin and hair.

During the actual **menstruation stage** (if no egg has become fertilized and implanted), all other hormone levels drop, and prostaglandin levels rise. If you can understand the different parts of your cycle, it can make your life a lot easier. You can adjust your diet, skincare routine, and physical activities to avoid any disruptions, such as bloating and skin issues.

The Four Stages of Menstruation

You may have thought that menstruation was just a few days of period bleeding...

NOPE!

As it was lightly outlined in the previous section, there are a total of four phases in the menstrual cycle: menstruation, the follicular phase, ovulation, and the luteal phase.

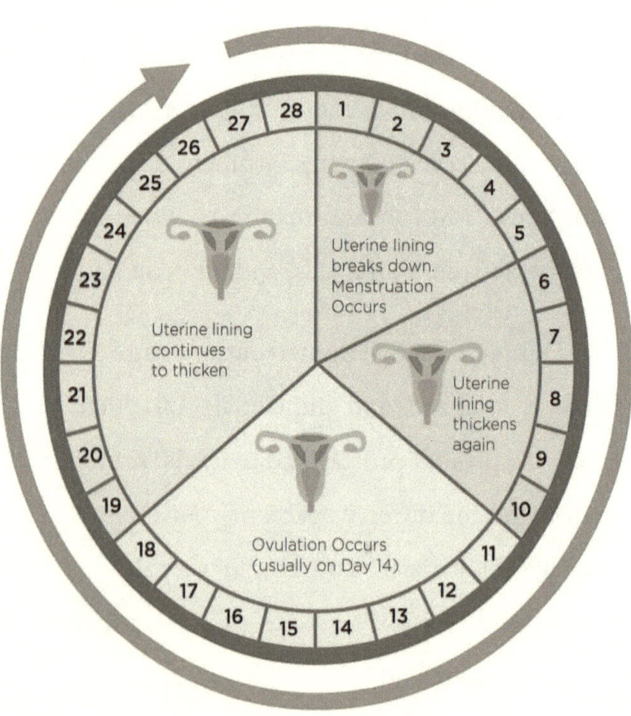

Menstrual Phase

The first phase of the menstrual cycle is the *menstrual phase*. In this stage, the inner lining of the uterine wall breaks down and sheds through the vagina. Menstrual blood contains blood, obviously; cells from the inner lining of the uterus, also known as endometrial cells, and mucus (BetterHealth, 2014).

<u>Fun Fact:</u> Most women have period stains in every pair of underwear they own, so don't feel bad if you have some too! But if you want to avoid stains, you can try wearing panty liners in between your periods.

Follicular Phase

The *follicular phase* overlaps with the menstruation phase, beginning on the first day of menstruation. Your brain plays a big part in this stage. The pituitary gland releases a follicle- stimulating hormone, or FSH (BetterHealth, 2014), which releases a follicle with an immature egg. This phase occurs typically between day ten and twenty-eight of the cycle. This process also signals the uterus to thicken to prepare for a baby (BetterHealth, 2014).

Ovulation

Ovulation arises when a mature egg is released from the ovary, which generally transpires mid-cycle and approximately two weeks before menstruation starts. It triggers within two days of the release of GnRH, LH, and FSH hormones (BetterHealth, 2014). The egg has a lifespan of about twenty-four hours unless fertilized by a sperm, in which case it would then implant and grow into a fetus.

If your goal is to become pregnant, a good strategy is to track your cycle. By tracking your cycle, you can be aware of your peak fertility days and engage in intercourse during those days.

Luteal Phase

The final phase is the *luteal phase*. During ovulation, the egg remains held inside a follicle (which looks like a bubble) until ovulation. At this point, the egg bursts out of the follicle. The ruptured part of the follicle remains attached to the surface of the uterus for about two weeks (BetterHealth, 2014).

This ruptured follicle is called the **corpus luteum**. It releases *progesterone*, which thickens the lining of the uterus in preparation for implantation (American Pregnancy Association [APA], 2019). The corpus luteum will produce the hormone progesterone for the next twelve to sixteen days of the cycle, which makes up the luteal phase. If the egg becomes fertilized, then progesterone will continue to be produced by the corpus luteum until the pregnancy has developed far enough for the placenta to take over (APA, 2019).

Menstrual cycle

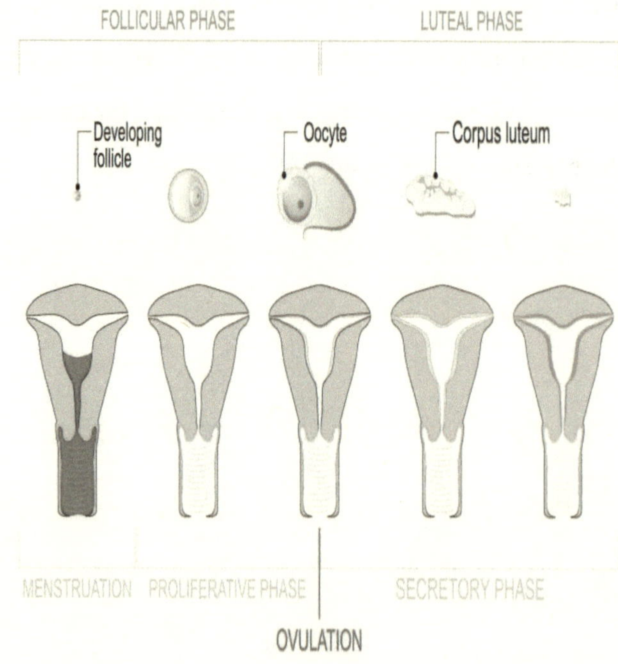

Vaginal Discharge

Vaginal discharge isn't usually the topic of choice when sitting down over coffee; although if you do choose to discuss women's health topics over coffee, props to you!

Every woman experiences vaginal discharge; it's completely normal. Not all vaginal discharge is quite the same, however. Your discharge can be a great indicator of your health or lack thereof. Infections can cause your discharge to change. If you see any concerning changes in your discharge, you should contact your doctor to discuss testing and treatment options.

So, let's get down to everything you ever wanted to know about vaginal discharge.

Vaginal Discharge Colours and What They Mean

Our bodies are amazing in sending us signals to help indicate our health and well-being. The different colours and consistencies of your vaginal discharge are your body's way of telling you if something is right or wrong.

So, don't be afraid to examine your discharge and talk to your doctor about it if anything feels worrying.

White Discharge

Generally speaking, white discharge is normal, particularly at the beginning or end of your menstrual cycle (Ellis, 2018). White discharge is usually the standard colour. However, it can also signal a yeast infection if it is thick and has a cottage cheese-like consistency, and especially if accompanied by itching. If you are experiencing this type of discharge, then you should consult your doctor and ask about treatment options. There are many over-the-counter options for treating a yeast infection.

Clear and Watery Discharge

This discharge is natural and the colour and consistency that you want. It is perfectly normal and will likely occur during most of the month. If this discharge bothers you and you feel self-conscious about it, you can wear a thin panty liner to protect your underwear. It may also come out a little heavier after working out (Ellis, 2018).

Clear and Stretchy Discharge

This discharge indicates that you are ovulating. Ovulation discharge is mostly transparent with a mucus-like consistency rather than a watery consistency. If you are trying to track your ovulation and menstruation, make sure you are also taking note of the kinds of vaginal discharge you are experiencing. (Ellis, 2018).

Yellowish or Greenish Discharge

This discharge is *bad*. If you experience a thick, yellowish or greenish discharge (that may or may not have a funky smell), you may have a **sexually transmitted infection** (STI) known as **trichomoniasis** (Ellis, 2018). If you are experiencing this kind of discharge, you should see your **obstetrics and gynaecology professional** (OB-GYN) as soon as possible.

Causes of Different Types of Vaginal Discharge

While it is normal for your body to expel vaginal discharge, colour, consistency, and smell can tell you a great deal about your overall and reproductive health. Generally, your vaginal discharge should be pale white, clear and mucus-like. If you experience other types of discharge, you likely have an imbalance of some kind in your genitals.

The production of vaginal discharge is your vagina's self-cleaning mechanism. Many things can lead to changes in your vaginal discharge: sexual intercourse, ovulation, birth control, exercise, and emotional stress are some examples. But you must watch out for abnormalities in your discharge in case of infection.

Trichomoniasis

I mentioned this kind of infection earlier when I discussed how vaginal discharge could also change to a yellowish or greenish colour.

Trichomoniasis is a type of **STI**, meaning that it is usually spread through sexual intercourse. STIs move through vaginal fluids, semen, or blood. A person can contract them through the use of dirty needles or open cuts that become infected. Tattoo artists and medical professionals are required to switch needles every time they give someone a tattoo or a shot. These precautions help to reduce the potential spreading of STIs. (Centre for Young Women's Health [CYWH], 2017).

In addition to a yellow or greenish-coloured discharge, there is also a foul odour that comes along with it. Women who have contracted trichomoniasis can also experience pain, itching, and inflammation. However, some women are **asymptomatic**, meaning they don't experience any symptoms (Ellis, 2018).

Trichomoniasis is diagnosed through **urinalysis** (a urine test). The condition is treated with an oral dose of metronidazole or tinidazole (types of antibiotics; Mayo Clinic Staff, 2018). If diagnosed, medical professionals suggest that both you and your partner undergo treatment and abstain from sexual intercourse until the infection has cleared. If left untreated, trichomoniasis can last for months to years, so if you ever experience these symptoms, definitely do not hesitate to see your doctor.

Bacterial Vaginosis

A rather common bacterial infection that many women experience, **bacterial vaginosis** is when excessive bacteria grow in the vagina. While the colour of the vaginal discharge may not drastically change, it can have a strong odour or "fishy" smell. Some women might experience a discharge that is thin, grey, white, or even greenish, accompanied by vaginal itching or burning during urination (Mayo Clinic Staff, 2019). Women are more likely to contract bacterial vaginosis if they receive oral sex or engage in intercourse with multiple partners (Ellis, 2018).

Bacterial vaginosis can be diagnosed through a pelvic exam, taking a sample of the vaginal secretions, or testing vaginal pH levels (Mayo Clinic Staff, 2019). Bacterial vaginosis can also be treated with oral medications. As this infection only occurs within a vagina, only partners with a vagina are required to test for bacterial vaginosis.

Yeast Infections

Yeast infections are also a widespread occurrence

that will cause abnormal vaginal discharge. **Yeast infections** are often categorized by burning, itching, and cottage cheese-like discharge. While it is reasonable to have yeast in the vagina, there are some situations where its growth can get out of control and cause an infection (Ellis, 2018).

Women often experience yeast infections as a side effect of pregnancy, diabetes, birth control pills, stress, and prolonged use of antibiotics. It is rather easy to self-diagnose a yeast infection and seek over-the-counter treatments. If you are unsure if you have a yeast infection, you should consult your doctor. They can perform a pelvic exam and test your vaginal discharge. Treatment can include antifungal vaginal cream or a single-dose oral medication (Mayo Clinic Staff, 2019).

Gonorrhoea and Chlamydia

Gonorrhoea and chlamydia are two common STIs, which result in a discoloured vaginal discharge that is greenish, yellowish, or cloudy (Ellis, 2018). Gonorrhoea can affect both men and women, most often affecting the cervix in women. Women are usually asymptomatic when it comes to gonorrhoea. If you experience symptoms such as increased vaginal discharge, pain while urinating, spotting after sexual intercourse, painful intercourse, abdominal or pelvic pain, you should consult your doctor (Mayo Clinic Staff, 2019).

Gonorrhoea can affect other parts of the body as well, including the rectum, and have symptoms similar to haemorrhoids. It can also affect the eyes and cause eye pain and sensitivity. It can manifest in the throat and result in swollen lymph nodes and joints, resulting in **septic arthritis** (Mayo Clinic Staff, 2019). Doctors can diagnose gonorrhoea with a urine test or swabbing an infected area. There are also home testing kits available in-store and online, and a rather simple round of antibiotics administered by your doctor should clear things up. Your partner should also get tested and treated for the STI to prevent further infection (Mayo Clinic Staff, 2019).

Chlamydia is another frequent STI that appears asymptomatic; 90% of women and 70% of men don't even realize they have it (Seladi-Schulman, 2019). While there are not many issues with having chlamydia short-term, there are some severe health complications that can arise if left untreated. Unprotected vaginal and oral sex are the leading causes of chlamydia, and symptoms can manifest via discoloured vaginal discharge. The infection rate among young women between the ages of fifteen and twenty-four are the highest reported, and the Centres for Disease Control (CDC) recommends that sexually active young women get tested annually (Seladi-Schulman, 2019).

It can often take several weeks for chlamydia symptoms to appear. Some of the most common symptoms include painful intercourse, discoloured vaginal discharge, burning during urination, pain in the lower abdomen, bleeding or spotting between periods, and inflammation of the cervix. In some rare cases, the infection can result in a condition called pelvic inflammatory disease (PID), which is a medical emergency that affects the fallopian tubes. PID symptoms include fever, severe pelvic pain, nausea, and abnormal bleeding between periods (Seladi-Schulman, 2019). If caught early enough, antibiotics should do the trick and have you back to normal in no time.

Chapter Summary

Your menstrual cycle lasts the entire month and not just the time you spend bleeding. There are four different stages: menstruation, the follicular phase, ovulation, and the luteal phase.

During the menstrual phase, you experience menstrual bleeding as your uterine lining sheds. The follicular phase starts on the first day of menstruation and releases a follicle with an immature egg. Ovulation occurs when a mature egg is released. Finally, the luteal phase is when the ruptured follicle hangs out in the uterus until it is discarded during menstruation.

Many factors can affect the length of a woman's menstrual cycle. These include alcohol consumption, smoking, drug use, body weight, physical activity, medical conditions, etc.

Vaginal discharge consists of the fluid and cells that are dispelled from the body. This discharge comes through the vagina and varies in colour and consistency. The colours and consistency of vaginal discharge can include white, smooth, mucus-like, cottage cheese-like, greenish, stretchy, brown, bloody, thick, yellowish, watery, and foul-smelling.

Changes in vaginal discharge can indicate bacterial infections or diseases such as trichomoniasis, bacterial vaginosis, yeast infections, gonorrhoea, or chlamydia.

While there are many reasons that vaginal discharge can change, you should use it to help indicate your reproductive health. If you have any concerns about your discharge, you should consult with your doctor.

In the next chapter, we are going to cover PMS, how to understand the symptoms of PMS and PMT, PMDD, and some tips on how to manage your PMS symptoms.

CHAPTER FOUR – WHAT IS PMS?

The term **PMS**, or premenstrual syndrome, is often synonymous with *that time of the month*. Those who are unaware of what PMS is, merely view it as a woman being short-tempered and unapproachable during menstruation. While this might be true for some ladies, PMS has a lot more to do with your cycle than just being irritable.

In this chapter, we are going to cover what PMS and PMT are and how not all ladies suffer from PMT or PMS symptoms. We will also cover the physical and psychological symptoms of PMS and PMT, tips on how to manage PMS, what PMDD is, and when you should seek medical advice.

An Easy to Understand Medical Definition of PMS and PMT

Many women experience PMS at various times of the month, often right around when they're supposed to menstruate. It affects all women differently and can be much more severe in some than in others. Premenstrual tension, or PMT, has similar symptoms compared to PMS. Although each woman is different, there are many common symptoms that women face when experiencing PMS and PMT.

Some medical treatments for PMS and PMT include **hormonal therapy** (birth control), **cognitive behavioural therapy** (CBT), and antidepressants. These treatments should be a last resort. Doctors generally only consider these treatment options for the following reasons. Either you are unable to function in society, or you tried all other possible lifestyle changes, and they did not work.

The main reason women experience PMS and PMT is because of hormonal changes. As stated previously, every woman is distinct from each other.

Some woman women may experience severe PMS symptoms; others will have very mild to no symptoms at all (NHS, 2018). It is more common for certain groups of women to experience signs of PMS. These groups include women who have already had children, those who don't exercise regularly, eat an unhealthy diet, and have high levels of stress (Home Health UK. 2017).

Fun Fact: As recently as the 1950s, women were diagnosed with something called *female hysteria*, with symptoms such as outbursts, irritability, anxiety, and increased sexual desire (Dusenbery, 2017). *Hysterika* is Greek for "uterus" and was known as a "disease of women;" it was used to describe all kinds of different problems that women faced in terms of their bodies (Dusenbery, 2017; Traniello, n.d.). Historians may argue, but luckily, the belief that a genital massage was the cure is likely just a myth (Meyer & Fetters, 2018).

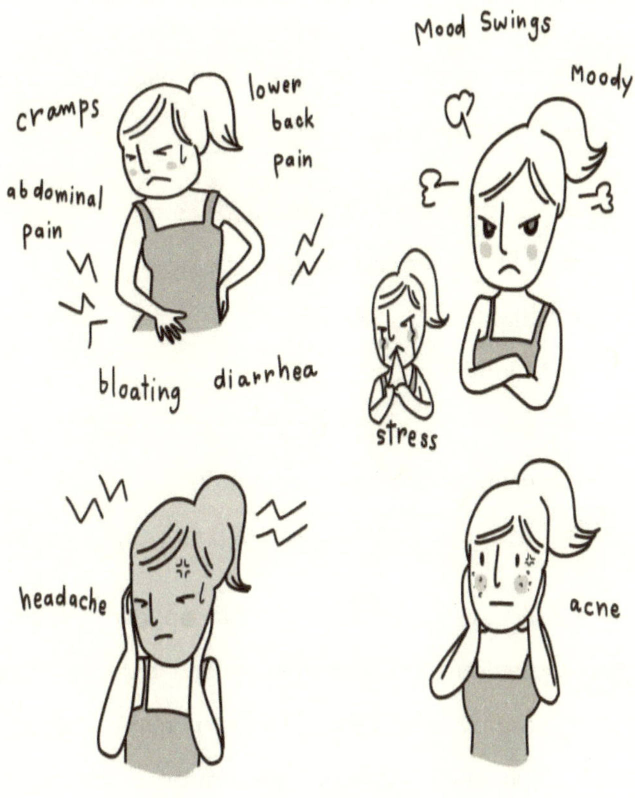

PMS SYMPTOMS
Premenstrual Syndrome

The Physical Symptoms Of PMS And PMT

Symptoms of PMS and PMT can manifest into many physical symptoms:

- Tender or swollen breasts.
- Headaches and stomach cramps.
- Skin and hair issues.
- Clumsiness.
- Food cravings or loss of appetite; weight gain/bloating; fluid retention.
- Insomnia; trouble sleeping; fatigue,

Generally, symptoms of PMS appear a few days before the start of menstruation and tend to decrease once bleeding has begun. However, many women will still experience physical discomforts during their menstruation as well, to be precise, the dreaded *stomach issues*.

Try to record when you are experiencing symptoms so you can estimate when to expect them in your next menstrual cycle. This practice can help you to better prepare for PMS symptoms and know if you should have any heating packs or ibuprofen to hand.

The Psychological Symptoms of PMS and PMT

Menstrual hormones mess with our brains just as much as they mess with our bodies. Even the most level-headed woman can let PMS get the best of her. Some of the psychological side effects of PMS and PMT include:

- An increase in sex drive.

- Mood swings - irritability, aggression, depression, mania.

- Feeling upset for no apparent reason.

While some women might be a little moodier during this time of the month, others can seem like they are on the edge of a nervous breakdown. When we experience these hormonal changes, it can sometimes be too much to bear. For this reason, you should avoid making any big life decisions while you are experiencing disruptive psychological PMS symptoms.

Not All Ladies Suffer from PMT or PMS

While some ladies experience intense PMS symptoms, others hardly experience any. If you are one of the unlucky ladies to experience severe PMS symptoms, you might think it's normal and that everyone has similar symptoms. This belief is not entirely true; there are some lucky women out there, even without the ideal lifestyle adjustments, who don't experience PMS.

It's relatively tricky to tell how many women suffer from PMS, as the medical definition is rather vague, and PMS tends to be vastly underreported. There are not many medical studies on PMS, and the ones that are published are somewhat unreliable and include a very narrow demographic.

There are many physical or psychological symptoms, and several of them are linked. For example, you might experience *poor sleep* as a result of *feeling bloated*, thus be more *irritable* the next day. As there are numerous PMS symptoms, it can be difficult to tell if you are experiencing PMS, merely having a bad day, or if there are other factors at play.

Tips and Tricks to Managing Your PMS Symptoms

There are tons of lifestyle changes you can make to help minimize the symptoms associated with PMS and PMT. Even though working out may be the last thing you want to do with terrible stomach cramps, it can be beneficial. You might not want to run a marathon; but brisk walking, jogging, or even swimming are all great forms of light exercise. These exercises help your brain to release endorphins which minimize the physical pain you're feeling. So, remember next time you are laying on the couch and feeling like you are going to die — you should get up and take a walk. Trust me; it will you feel so much better. Not to mention, fresh air is always great for you.

When many women experience PMS, chocolate and ice cream are the only things they want to eat (believe me, we have all been there!). Dieticians believe that this sudden increase in cravings may be because the volume of cortisol (a stress hormone) in our bodies rises while the amount of serotonin (a mood regulator hormone) decreases. On top of that, our blood sugar levels also decrease. With all of these hormonal changes, something in our bodies tells us that we need some way to lower our stress levels and make us feel better. This usually leads us to want to eat unhealthy foods like ice cream and chocolate (Lama, 2018).

While it is perfectly fine to indulge here and there, moderation is key. Eating a healthy, balanced diet will help to minimize skin breakouts, feelings of nausea, and bloating. Even though our bodies may be craving something else, it is healthier food that will make you feel better. Think fresh, light meals, and lots of water.

Sleep is also crucial while you are experiencing PMS symptoms. It might be challenging to get a good night's sleep during menstruation. There are some ways to make yourself comfortable at night. These include having a warm milky (or vegan alternative) drink before bed or taking a hot water bottle into bed with you. These simple steps will help you to gain a solid seven to eight hours of sleep per night. A satisfying sleep will help you to feel rested and mitigate some of the physical symptoms that go along with PMS.

It seems that any situation can get the best of you when you are experiencing PMS, no matter how much you may try to control it. You were running late for work, and someone parked in your parking spot, well, let's take a deep br—

THE WORLD IS ENDING!

PMS and PMT rage can appear out of nowhere. Try to minimize your stress by practising yoga and meditation, so that when tense situations do arise, you will be better equipped to handle them.

If you don't want to see your general practitioner for your PMS symptoms, then try some over-the-counter medications. Painkillers such as ibuprofen and paracetamol can help ease the physical discomforts of your menstrual cycle.

You can also try upping your vitamin and mineral intake during times of PMS. Vitamin B6, magnesium, and calcium can also help reduce symptoms associated with PMS. Some women likewise find relief from breast tenderness and other PMS symptoms by taking the recommended daily allowance of evening primrose oil (Home Health UK, 2017).

Self-care is essential for all of us. Women often put it to the wayside, especially if they are a mother. Many women tend to put everyone else's needs before their own. Whether or not it is your time of the month and you are experiencing PMS symptoms, you should take time for yourself. Taking time can mean self-care through meditation, developing a good daily skincare routine, or even sitting down with a glass of wine and a good book. Find something that will help you to relax and revitalize yourself.

Remember to keep a diary of your symptoms. A journal will help you pinpoint your symptoms and if certain things will trigger worse symptoms. For example, you had a craving for ice cream but then felt bloated afterwards. Perhaps during your menstrual cycle, you are more sensitive to dairy products, so next time try a non-dairy alternative and see if you experience the same side effects. Keeping a diary can also be beneficial for your mental health. You might not always have someone to talk to about how you are feeling; writing in a journal can help to understand your emotions during your menstrual cycle.

Some of the things you should avoid when you are experiencing PMS (and as a general health rule) are smoking and drinking too much alcohol. While it may help relieve some stress in the short-term, it's not going to provide you with any long-term physical or mental benefits. In short: maybe wine, but not too much wine.

It's also necessary to avoid foods that are high in sodium, as this leads to more water retention and bloated feeling. While exercise is generally beneficial, don't overdo it if you are experiencing severe PMS symptoms, since this will likely only make them worse.

If you have tried all of these lifestyle changes and nothing seems to be working, then it might be time to contact your general practitioner. If you find that your PMS and PMT symptoms are drastically affecting your daily life, it's a good idea to contact your practitioner. There could potentially be some underlying issues that need further investigation and diagnosis (NHS, 2018). A symptoms diary can also help you share information with your doctor that you might have otherwise forgotten.

As discussed, many women experience severe PMS symptoms — but many of them may not realize they are experiencing **premenstrual dysphoric disorder** or PMDD. If you are experiencing severe PMS symptoms, you should consult your practitioner with a record of your symptoms in case you are suffering from this disorder.

What is Premenstrual Dysphoric Disorder (PMDD)?

PMDD is like PMS on steroids. It is very similar to PMS but is much worse and should be diagnosed by your general practitioner. PMDD can cause severe irritability, depression, and or anxiety a week or two before your period is supposed to start. While symptoms generally subside about two to three days before the start of your period, you might need some medication to help alleviate these symptoms.

PMDD is caused by a drop in hormone levels after ovulation occurs. Many women who experience PMDD also experience anxiety and depression in addition to more severe PMS symptoms. Symptoms of PMDD include:

- Uncontrollable irritability or anger; out of control.
- Symptoms correlated to depression, such as suicidal thoughts, low energy and issues. sleeping,

    lack of stimulating daily activities and relationships.

- Intense feelings of tension, anxiety, sadness; panic attacks; crying often.
- Drastic mood swings.
- Problems focusing or thinking.
- Binge eating; strong food cravings.
- More intense physical symptoms.

Just as with PMS, researchers have not pinpointed the cause of PMDD but rather attribute it to the hormonal changes that transpire during the menstrual cycle. One aspect might be that some women are more sensitive to the change in serotonin levels that others, which can cause the more severe symptoms that lead to PMDD.

Your general practitioner can diagnose PMDD by going through your health history and doing a physical exam. For this purpose, again, is where a journal will come in handy. Write down everything you can think of that is related to your menstrual cycle. You should include how you feel both physically and emotionally, the food you eat and how your mood is fluctuating throughout the day.

Depending on the treatment course that your doctor deems appropriate, you could either get prescribed antidepressants, birth control, over-the-counter medications, or prescribed stress-management techniques. It is also wise to take a look at your eating and lifestyle habits to determine if making changes there will help with your symptoms.

When to Seek Medical Advice

You can treat a lot of PMS and PMDD symptoms with over-the-counter medications and lifestyle changes, but there are times when you should seek medical advice. For example, if you are feeling extremely upset with some inclinations toward self-harm, you should seek out the help of a medical professional (Planned Parenthood, 2019).

If you experience any of the following symptoms, you should contact your doctor *immediately*. These include a fever of 102° Fahrenheit or higher, severe muscle aches, diarrhoea, vomiting, dizziness, a rash that looks comparable to a sunburn, a sore throat, and bloodshot eyes. These are all potential signs of **toxic shock syndrome**, which can cause severe long-term health issues or even death if left untreated.

If you continue to experience severe PMS symptoms, then you should also contact your doctor. This will allow your doctor to rule out other issues that may or may not be related to your reproductive health.

Chapter Summary

Many people associate PMS, or premenstrual syndrome, with "that time of the month." While some women can undoubtedly be irritable while experiencing PMS and PMT symptoms, there is a lot more to PMS than just being in a bad mood. With over 150 PMS symptoms, there are a lot of issues that can arise during menstruation, including but not limited to: weight gain, irritation, aggression, stomach cramps, food cravings, and emotional mood swings.

Most women can get relief from PMS and PMT symptoms with some simple lifestyle changes. However, others might need a little extra help, which include hormonal therapy, cognitive behavioural therapy, and antidepressants.

Many women experience PMS and PMT symptoms due to hormonal changes and poor lifestyle choices. PMS symptoms should only last for a few days before menstruation starts; however, every woman is unique and may experience PMS symptoms differently. For many reasons, it is a good idea to keep a record of your menstrual cycle and your associated symptoms. This way, if you need to seek the advice of a medical professional, you have a written history of your symptoms.

For some women, PMS causes a lot of suffering; for others, they are entirely asymptomatic. If you are unlucky and experience more severe PMS and PMT symptoms, you can make lifestyle choices that should help to improve your symptoms. Some simple lifestyle changes that you can start to incorporate are:

- Light cardio and strength training.
- Eating a healthy, balanced diet.
- Sleeping well and taking it easy.
- Yoga and meditation for stress relief.
- Painkillers.

- Consuming more vitamins and natural supplements.

PMDD is like PMS or PMT but accompanied by more severe anxiety, depressive, and/or physical symptoms. PMDD should be diagnosed by your general practitioner and might often require prescription medication.

If you experience any severe physical symptoms, such as a fever or a rash that looks like a sunburn, you should contact your doctor immediately. There may be a chance that you are suffering from toxic shock syndrome.

In the next chapter, we are going to take a more in-depth look at the principal physical, and psychological symptoms women experience during menstruation. Also, we will focus on the causes of painful periods, and why some women experience excessively heavy periods. Finally, we will discuss endometriosis.

CHAPTER FIVE – WHY DO I FEEL DIFFERENT DURING MY PERIOD?

It is common for women to feel different during their periods in one way or another. Some women might not experience any pain during their periods and menstrual cycles, while others want to lay in the fetal position with a heating pad all day.

In this chapter, we are going to cover the potential causes of painful periods, the roots of heavy periods, endometriosis, and the causes and treatments for endometriosis.

We have talked a lot about the different physical and psychological symptoms that women experience when on their periods. There are a whole host of symptoms, both physical and psychological that women experience when they are menstruating. It's not uncommon for women to confuse PMS and PMT with early pregnancy signs. And many women also experience painful periods.

Causes of Painful Periods

Painful periods, or **dysmenorrhea**, is pain associated with menstruation. Pain during periods is the most commonly reported disorder related to menstruation. More than half of all menstruating women will experience period pain. Period pain tends to last for between one to two days each month (American College of Obstetricians and Gynaecologists [ACOG], 2015).

There are two principal types of dysmenorrhea: *primary* and *secondary*. The primary kind is caused from having menstrual cramps, whereas the secondary kind appears later in life and is caused by a disorder in the reproductive system and tends to worsen over time (ACOG, 2015).

The pain caused by *primary dysmenorrhea* is from the release of prostaglandins, made in the lining of the uterus. Primary dysmenorrhea starts when a girl has her first period and tends to lessen either after childbirth or with age. Pain from *secondary dysmenorrhea* is caused by conditions such as endometriosis, adenomyosis, and fibroids (ACOG, 2015).

Your general practitioner can diagnosis you with primary or secondary dysmenorrhea with either a pelvic exam or using an ultrasound machine. Doctors treat dysmenorrhea in much the same way as PMS and PMDD symptoms; treatments can include hormonal medication, over-the-counter pain relievers, or lifestyle changes like eating healthy and exercising. In extreme cases of secondary dysmenorrhea, your doctor may suggest surgery to provide you with relief (ACOG, 2015)

Causes of Heavy Periods

Heavy periods, also known as **menorrhagia**, often accompany dysmenorrhea. If you are experiencing heavy bleeding, it does not mean that there is anything wrong with you. It can, however, affect you both physically and emotionally (NHS Direct Wales, 2019). Every person's menstruation is different, with varying levels of pain and volume. What one woman feels is a heavy period may be light compared to someone else. The average amount of blood that a woman menstruates is thirty to forty millilitres, with a heavy flow defined as sixty or more millilitres (NHS Direct Wales, 2019).

If you have been getting your period for some time, you should know what is considered uniquely normal and heavy for you. There are many signs you can look out for to determine if you are experiencing an unusually heavy menstrual cycle. These signs include the need to use an exceptionally high number of pads or tampons, experiencing heavy bleeding through your clothing or bedding (otherwise known as flooding), or needing to use tampons and pads at the same time.

Fun Fact: On average, women go through 12,000 to 15,000 pads, tampons, and panty liners in their lifetime of menstruation.

While many women experience heavy periods for seemingly no reason, certain medical conditions can cause more excessive bleeding.

- **Polycystic Ovary Syndrome (PCOS)** — a disorder in which a woman's hormone levels are out of balance, producing higher-than-normal amounts of androgens (male hormones) and causing skips in menstrual periods and much heavier periods.

- **Pelvic Inflammatory Disease (PID)** — an infection in a woman's reproductive system that leads to pelvic pain and excess bleeding between periods or after sex.

- **Fibroids** — a benign growth in or around the womb leading to heavy or painful periods.

- **Endometriosis.**

- **Adenomyosis** — when womb tissue becomes embedded in the lining of the womb, causing heavy bleeding.

- **Hypothyroidism** — an underactive thyroid gland that doesn't produce enough hormones, leading to excessive fatigue, weight gain, and depression.

- **Polyps (cervical and endometrial)** — benign growths on the inside of the womb or cervix.

- Cancer of the womb (rare).

- Inserting an IUD can cause heavier bleeding the first three to six months after insertion.

- Anticoagulant medication.

- Some medications used for chemotherapy.

As you can see, many things can cause excessive or irregular bleeding. If you are concerned with heavy bleeding, then you should contact your general practitioner. They should be able to diagnose any issues you are having with a pelvic exam or give you a blood test to determine any underlying issues.

If your heavy periods are uncomfortable, but not affecting your everyday life, then a simple lifestyle change might improve your situation. However, if you need a prescribed treatment for your heavy menstrual bleeding, then hormonal therapy might be necessary.

Journaling your periods and symptoms will come in handy here. Keep a journal of when you are experiencing heavy bleeding and any related symptoms. Jot down things like how long your periods last, how often you have to change your pad or tampon, if you are experiencing flooding, if you are bleeding between periods or after sex, if you are experiencing pelvic or abdominal pain, if you are already taking birth control and if so, what kind, and any other related symptoms or lifestyle factors. You should also discuss any family history that you know of in case there are genetic factors at play.

Endometriosis

The **endometrium** is a membrane made up of mucosal tissue that lines the uterus and helps cover and protect the developing fetus (Cornforth, 2019). **Endometriosis** then is "the presence of endometrial-like tissue outside the uterus, which induces a chronic, inflammatory reaction" (Kennedy et al., 2005). Women of reproductive age are the majority affected by endometriosis. It is not limited to ethnicity or social class and can have an impact on physical and mental health, as well as overall well-being. It is imperative that if you experience heavy bleeding or other types of abnormal menstrual symptoms, to speak with your doctor. Don't discount your symptoms as just period pain.

Endometriosis generally appears as lesions on the ovaries that look like powder-burns and are black, dark brown or bluish. The extent of the disease can vary widely, and it can manifest into a few small lesions and then into large ovarian cysts (Kennedy et al., 2005). It can be difficult to diagnose endometriosis just from describing symptoms alone. Doctors will often need to make further tests, as symptoms often overlap with other conditions such as PID and irritable bowel syndrome (Kennedy et al., 2005). Diagnosis often includes a visual inspection of the pelvis via a laparoscopy. Several of the remedies for endometriosis include over-the-counter drugs, hormonal treatments, GnRH treatment, and surgical treatments.

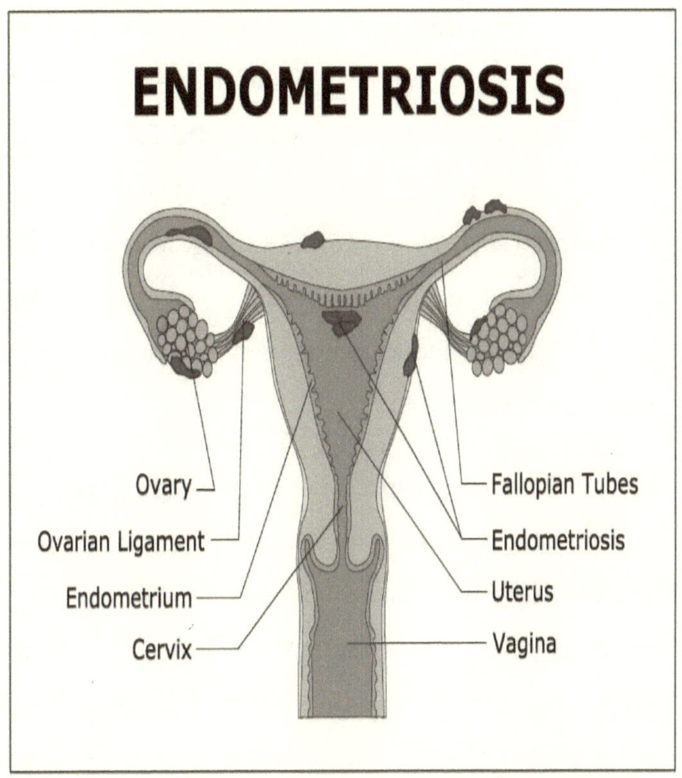

It is common for women to take *non-steroidal anti-inflammatory drugs*, or NSAIDs, to help reduce pain associated with endometriosis. However, you should be aware that taking NSAIDs can affect your body in other ways. If you take them mid-cycle, they can stop or decrease ovulation. Furthermore, if you have them too often, they can cause stomach ulcers (Kennedy et al., 2005).

Hormonal treatments via birth control can also help to reduce endometriosis-associated pain. If the functioning of the ovaries is suppressed for six months, it can help to reduce pain drastically. Specific hormonal treatments such as danazol, COC, gestrinone, GnRH agonists, and medroxyprogesterone acetate all work equally well for reducing endometriosis-associated pain (Kennedy et al., 2005).

If the doctor suspects the disease is progressing and hormonal treatment is insufficient, they may order a **laparoscopy** be carried out. A laparoscopy is an examination in which the surgeon looks at the pelvic organs to see if endometriosis is indeed present; if so, the surgeon will begin the procedure to treat it. Depending on your age and the severity of your endometriosis, your next procedures could vary. It is vital that you report suspected endometriosis, as the later you treat it, the worse your pain could be and the higher your chances of infertility (Healthwise Staff, 2018). Please don't be afraid to talk to your doctor if you feel you might have endometriosis. This could help you avoid undergoing invasive testing and then needing to have a separate surgery (Kennedy et al., 2005).

Chapter Summary

Periods are frustrating. You can be feeling great, then boom — your period is about to hit, and you're experiencing debilitating symptoms that can affect your daily life.

There are many medical reasons as to why a woman would experience heavy or painful bleeding. These are most commonly due to menstrual cramping, endometriosis, adenomyosis, and fibroids. Many women also experience menorrhagia, which is often accompanied by painful periods.

If you think that you might have any of the conditions outlined in this chapter, you should contact your general practitioner to get a pelvic exam or blood test. If you experience heavy periods that aren't affecting your everyday life, perhaps a few simple lifestyle choices could help give you some relief.

Many women of reproductive age have endometriosis, causing heavy bleeding as well as difficulty in conceiving. Endometriosis can be treated via over-the-counter medications, hormonal treatments, GnRH hormone, and if necessary, surgery.

In the next chapter, we are going to talk about irregular periods, why you need to bleed between periods and causes for a period to stop. Also, we will discuss how to tell if you are perimenopausal and when you should seek out medical advice for concerning conditions.

CHAPTER SIX – WHAT HAPPENS WHEN YOUR PERIODS STOP?

What a regular period is to one woman is likely entirely abnormal for another. The thought of not having to bleed from your vagina each month might sound great to some women. Conversely, the underlying issues as to why your period stops might not outweigh the convenience of forgoing tampons.

In this chapter, we are going to cover irregular periods, why bleeding can still occur between your periods and amenorrhea. Then we will look at how to determine if you are perimenopausal, and when you seek advice from a medical professional for concerning conditions.

Irregular Periods

Several things can cause irregular periods, known as oligomenorrhea, from medical conditions to lack of calories. When you are just starting to get your period, and you are on the verge of ending your period, it is normal for it to be inconsistent. Not every woman experiences a twenty-eight day cycle with "normal" bleeding for four to seven days.

Some women can set a clock by when they get their periods. Other women need to carry pads or tampons because they never know when menstruation will start. There are a whole host of reasons as to why you might be experiencing irregular periods, including but not limited to:

- Medications; hormonal birth control.
- High or low body weight; excessive exercise; not eating enough calories.
- Hormonal imbalances; stress; eating disorders.
- Pregnancy; breastfeeding; perimenopause.
- Medical issues such as thyroid issues, uterine fibroids, endometriosis, cervical or endometrial cancer, PCOS.
- Endometriosis; cervical or endometrial cancer.

If you are experiencing irregular periods and have

been sexually active, you might want to consider taking a pregnancy test. Even during pregnancy, some women can experience bleeding during what they would conclude as just another period. If you are pregnant, you will want to make an appointment with your obstetrics and gynaecology team for prenatal care.

Furthermore, if you are experiencing sharp abdominal pains, then you should consult with your doctor immediately. Whether you know you are pregnant or not, you might be experiencing a miscarriage or an ectopic pregnancy (Santos-Longhurst, 2018).

If you have given birth and are breastfeeding, you will likely not have much of a period, if at all. Breast milk is produced via the hormone prolactin, which suppresses reproductive hormones. This suppression of hormones means you will likely either have very light periods or no periods during the time you are breastfeeding. But be aware, you CAN still get pregnant even if your period doesn't arrive and you are breastfeeding. So, if you are not planning for another baby right away, you should consult your doctor on what birth control methods are best for you.

Certain medications, such as blood thinners, thyroid medications, epilepsy drugs, antidepressants, chemotherapy drugs, aspirin, and hormone replacement therapy can all cause your menstrual cycle to become irregular (Santos-Longhurst, 2018).

Excessive stress can also mess with your cycle. The brain controls your stress levels, as with the hormones that regulate your cycle. When you experience a lot of stress, it can interfere with the part of your brain that helps to regulate your cycle. You can reduce your stress through self-care practices such as meditation, yoga, exercise, aromatherapy, cutting back on caffeine, laughing, practising mindfulness, and of course, having an orgasm.

Fun Fact: Orgasms can help reduce period pain and make your cramps feel better by releasing pain-fighting neurotransmitters such as endorphins and oxytocin.

Female athletes often have irregular periods due to excessive physical exercise. Engaging in extreme physical activity interferes with the hormones that help to regulate your menstruation. It is not uncommon for marathon runners, gymnasts, dancers, and other athletes to miss or even stop menstruating, which is called **amenorrhea**. Depending on your fitness or fertility goals, you can quickly restore your periods by increasing your caloric intake to match your exercise exertion (Santos-Longhurst, 2018).

If you are rapidly losing weight or extremely restricting your calories, you may also experience amenorrhea. A drastic reduction in calories interferes with ovulation by not producing enough of the hormones required to make ovulation happen. Women that have a body mass index (BMI) below 18.5 are considered underweight and might also experience other symptoms like headaches, hair loss, and fatigue (Santos-Longhurst, 2018).

Just as with being underweight, being overweight can also impact the consistency of your menstrual cycle. It all comes down to hormones. Being overweight impacts insulin levels and hormones, which can interfere with the regulation of your menstrual cycle. Similar to rapid weight loss, you can also experience irregular periods if you gain weight too quickly. These two symptoms together can be a sign of hypothyroidism or polycystic ovarian syndrome (Santos-Longhurst, 2018). Your doctor can test for these with a simple blood test.

We discussed a lot about *endometriosis* in the previous chapter. Having an irregular period does not just mean missing a period here and there. It also refers to heavy bleeding, periods that last longer than normal and bleeding in between your periods. These symptoms, along with infertility, pain during or after sex, painful bowel movements, and gastrointestinal pains, can all be warning signs of endometriosis (Santos-Longhurst, 2018).

Uterine fibroids can also cause irregular periods. These are muscular tumours that form in the wall of the uterus. Not only are they painful, but uterine fibroids are generally benign and can range in size from an apple seed to a grapefruit. In addition to causing period irregularity, you may also experience painful and heavy periods. Other symptoms include lower back pain, pelvic pressure or pain, pain in your legs, and pain during sex. Fibroids are often managed and treated using over-the-counter medication (Santos-Longhurst, 2018).

Over 40% of women who experience irregularities in their menstrual cycle also have thyroid disorders. An underactive thyroid can lead to increased cramping and heavier and more prolonged periods. **Hypothyroidism** can also lead to sensitivity to cold, weight gain, and fatigue. The opposite disorder, **hyperthyroidism**, can lead to shorter and lighter periods, weight loss, heart palpitations, and anxiety (Santos-Longhurst, 2018).

Uterine fibroids

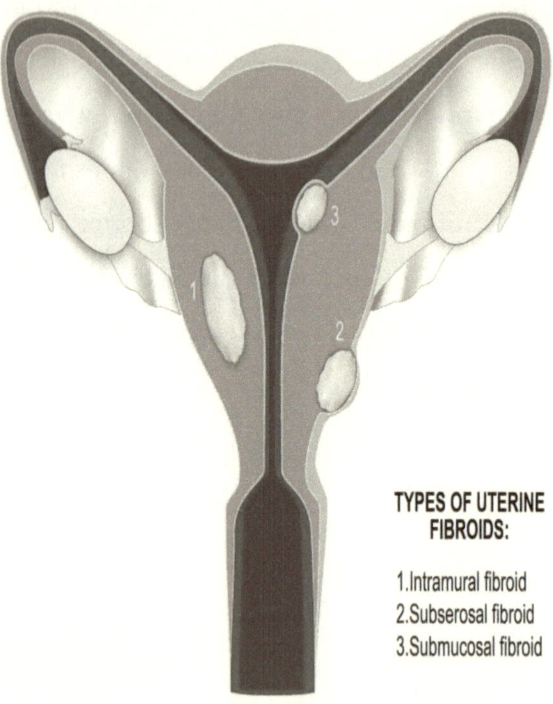

We touched a bit on PCOS previously, which can also lead to menstrual irregularity. Women who have PCOS can experience missed periods as well as heavy bleeding. In addition to these symptoms, PCOS can also cause infertility, weight gain or obesity, male-pattern baldness, and excess facial and body hair (Santos-Longhurst, 2018).

What you are taking for birth control can also play a significant factor in the regularity of your periods. Taking certain birth control pills can cause spotting in between your regular periods and much lighter periods. Many young women choose to take birth control pills as a way to regulate their periods and find relief from heavy and painful periods. IUDs, on the other hand, can cause much heavier periods (Santos-Longhurst, 2018).

Finally, if you are older (in your late 40s or so), then you might be experiencing irregular periods due to **perimenopause**. This term means your body is getting ready for the menopause and has begun the transition. Being perimenopausal can last anywhere from four to eight years. The perimenopausal phase starts to happen when your estrogen levels fluctuate. This causes irregular periods, hot flashes, night sweats, mood changes, difficulty sleeping, and vaginal dryness (Santos-Longhurst, 2018).

Why Do I Bleed Between Periods?

You may have been alarmed if you experienced bleeding between periods, but there is no cause for concern. Light blood flow, or spotting, between your regular menstrual bleeding, is entirely normal, and it's called **metrorrhagia** or **breakthrough bleeding**.

If you experience heavier bleeding between your regular periods, then there might be some underlying issues. These include an injury, hormonal changes, or other health concerns. Bleeding between your periods can happen any time between right before your period begins, or after it has already ended. Bleeding can range from light spotting to heavy bleeding, similar to a regular period.

Your complete menstrual cycle runs from the first day of one period to the first day of your next period. The period itself only lasts between five to seven days. But again, all women are different and may experience shorter or longer periods. Some people may experience periods lasting only two days if they are on a specific hormonal treatment. Just as with the cause of PMS symptoms, heavier bleeding, and irregular periods, there are many causes of metrorrhagia.

The use of hormonal contraceptives is a common cause of vaginal bleeding between periods (Sissons, 2018). Bleeding occurs for the first three months of using the contraceptive until the hormone levels balance out. If you experience heavier bleeding or irregular periods lasting longer than three months, you might want to seek medical attention. A doctor can check to see if there are other underlying issues and possibly change your contraception. Bleeding between periods can also happen if you are not taking your birth control correctly, such as skipping a pill. Emergency contraception, such as the morning-after pill, can (and should) also cause bleeding between your periods.

You can also experience bleeding between your periods as a result of pregnancy. Implantation bleeding is a sign that you have recently become pregnant and happens when a fertilized egg becomes attached to the uterine wall. Bleeding can also arise as a result of a miscarriage. A miscarriage can occur at any point during a known or unknown pregnancy. Furthermore, if you had a pregnancy that was terminated or aborted, you will also experience bleeding between your regular periods. If you have experienced this and your bleeding seems excessively heavy, you should consult your doctor (Sissons, 2018).

You can also experience spotting or bleeding between your period due to sexually transmitted infections (STIs). If you have had unprotected sex and are experiencing spotting or bleeding during sex, then it may be a sign of chlamydia.

Vaginal injuries may also be the cause of a bleeding or spotting incident between your periods. The skin inside your vagina is thin and delicate; it can easily tear during penetration, mainly if your vagina is dry. Many women experience vaginal dryness as a side effect poor arousal, changing hormonal levels, diabetes, or cancer treatment (Sissons, 2018). If your body is not producing enough of your natural vaginal lubrication, then you must have proper over-the-counter lubrication during sexual intercourse.

Women that are also perimenopausal will

generally experience bleeding in between their periods because their hormone levels become unstable at this stage (Sissons, 2018). After a woman has fully transitioned from being perimenopause to the menopause, their periods will stop. The **Menopause** is identified by a woman not having a period for one full year. Any vaginal bleeding after a woman has entered the menopause should be taken into concern as it could mean **uterine cancer**.

Polyps in the cervix or vagina can cause bleeding between periods as well. Generally, these will need to be removed, so they don't cause any further issues. Cervical cancer is another cause of vaginal bleeding between regular periods (Sissons, 2018). Early symptoms of cervical cancer include bleeding between periods, bleeding after sex, pain or discomfort during sex, and foul vaginal odour.

Why Have My Periods Stopped?

As I mentioned earlier, when your periods stop, it is referred to as amenorrhea. Amenorrhea is technically defined as when a girl has not menstruated by the time she reaches sixteen years old or when a woman has not menstruated for three months (Ellis, 2019). Some of the most common reasons women stop regularly having periods include pregnancy, breastfeeding, or the menopause. However, women may also stop menstruating due to lifestyle factors such as exercise level and body weight. In more rare cases, a woman's period might end due to reproductive issues and hormonal imbalances (Ellis, 2019). As with most reproductive health issues, you should contact your doctor if you are experiencing amenorrhea.

There are two different types of amenorrhea: primary and secondary. Primary is described above, whereas secondary is when a woman stops menstruating for more than three months.

While some women might still experience spotting while pregnant, many do not experience a period for a full nine months. Breastfeeding can also cause a woman to stop menstruating via the production of prolactin. Furthermore, the menopause is a common cause of amenorrhea in women of an older age. The menopause usually happens between the ages of forty-five to fifty-five, in which a woman can no longer become pregnant and stops producing eggs.

Fun Fact: In the 1700s, the menopause was seen by medical professionals as a deadly disease and was treated with things like leeches to the genitals and cervix and eclectic therapy, opium, and arsenic in the 1800s and 1900s (Sigurðardóttir, 2013). Those who studied medicine back then were mostly men, with little to no interest in learning about the female body to make proper, scientifically backed therapy (Di Noto, Newman, Wall, & Einstein, 2013).

Specific medication and genetic disorders can also cause amenorrhea. Using medicines that treat high blood pressure or chemotherapy, using antipsychotics or antidepressants, or suddenly stopping your birth control can all lead to periods ceasing. Some genetic disorders, such as Turner syndrome and Swyer syndrome, can cause girls to start menstruating later in life than others (Ellis, 2019).

Having too much or too little body fat and hormonal imbalances can also cause amenorrhea. Young athletic girls tend to have their periods later than their unathletic counterparts, as they tend to have lower levels of body fat. An excess of body fat can also lead to amenorrhea because the insulin levels are unstable. Hormonal imbalances, issues with thyroid, lower estrogen levels, and higher testosterone levels can all contribute to amenorrhea (Ellis, 2019).

In rare cases, physical and congenital disabilities can cause a late onset of menstruation or the absence of a period altogether (Ellis, 2019).

Perimenopause

People often don't realize that there are two stages to the menopause; we have a general understanding of the menopause, but not so much about the perimenopause. The perimenopause is the stage leading up to the menopause, which can last from a few years to a decade. Many women become premenopausal in their forties, but it can start as early as their thirties. During the perimenopause stage, your levels of estrogen will rise and fall, and you will experience shorter and irregular periods (Mayo Clinic Staff, 2017).

Some of the main symptoms of the perimenopause include:

- Irregular periods; vaginal and bladder problems, decreasing fertility; changes in sexual function.
- Issues sleeping and hot flashes.
- Mood changes.
- Loss of bone mass; change in cholesterol levels.

Perimenopausal symptoms are very similar to PMS symptoms, and many women might not even realize they are entering this change.

As your periods become more irregular, ovulation also becomes less predictable. As a result, the timing of your cycle is likely to change. Your periods might become shorter, longer, lighter or more substantial (Mayo Clinic Staff, 2017).

As with PMS symptoms, perimenopausal symptoms can all interlink to one another. Hot flashes and sleep issues are common among premenopausal women and are synonymous with the menopause. Hot flashes can vary in intensity, length, and frequency, and are uncomfortable and inconvenient. Sleep issues can arise from experiencing hot flashes or night sweats. Women might experience changes in their moods due to lack of sleep and related hormonal changes (Mayo Clinic Staff, 2017). Women might also experience depression during this stage, as they feel like they are losing a part of their womanhood.

A drop in estrogen can also cause vaginal issues, including decreased vaginal lubrication, elasticity, and tone, which can make sex uncomfortable (Mayo Clinic Staff, 2017). As if that isn't bad enough, decreased estrogen levels can also leave you more susceptible to urinary tract infections and vaginal infections. Try doing some simple Kegel exercises to keep your pelvic muscles strong. By keeping your pelvic muscles toned, you won't have to worry about peeing yourself every time you sneeze, cough, or laugh.

Believe me, none of this is fun.

During this time, your ovulation decreases, and so your ability to conceive also decreases. Depending on your goals, decreased ovulation could be either good or bad. If you are trying to conceive, you can still get pregnant for as long as you are having your period (I have worked with women who thought they were perimenopausal but were pregnant, so plan accordingly). If you are trying to avoid becoming pregnant, then you should continue to take birth control until you have not had a period for a full twelve months.

Considering the changes in your vaginal lubrication, electricity, and tone, in addition to numerous physical and emotional changes associated with the perimenopause, it's not uncommon for women to experience changes in their sexual desires. These changes are perfectly normal, and you should engage in conversation with your partner about any concerns that you have. However, if you had a healthy sex life before you started to experience perimenopausal symptoms, then it is likely not to change much (Mayo Clinic Staff, 2017).

Now would be an excellent time to start upping your calcium intake. With the decrease in estrogen levels, women tend to begin losing bone mass as well. When your bone density is decreasing faster than your body can replace it, you are at a higher risk of osteoporosis (Mayo

Clinic Staff, 2017). Your cholesterol levels are also subject to change due to your changing hormone and estrogen levels. During the perimenopause, your bad cholesterol (low-density lipoproteins; LDL) increases while your good cholesterol (high-density lipoproteins; HDL) decreases, which also puts you at a higher risk of heart disease (Mayo Clinic Staff, 2017).

Many of these symptoms can be mitigated with positive lifestyle adjustments, such as exercise, a healthy diet, and minimizing unhealthy habits.

When to Seek Medical Advice

You should never hesitate to seek out medical advice if you feel something is wrong. If you experience any perimenopausal symptoms interfering with your everyday life, then you should consult your general practitioner (particularly if you have high-risk factors). High-risk factors can include smoking, family history, cancer treatments, and hysterectomy.

The menopause generally occurs one to two years earlier for women who smoke (Mayo Clinic Staff, 2017). Furthermore, if you have a family history of women who have undergone early menopause, you might also be at risk for going through the menopause sooner than your peers. Chemotherapy, pelvic radiation therapy, and other cancer treatments can also cause an early onset of the menopause. Lastly, while you might not think that you would experience the menopause after having your uterus removed, if your ovaries are still intact, then you are going to experience the menopause. Your ovaries are what produce estrogen, which means you can still experience the menopause, often earlier than you usually would (Mayo Clinic Staff, 2017).

As I said before, one of the earliest signs of the perimenopause is the onset of irregular periods. If the only thing that has changed is the irregularity of your periods, then you shouldn't be concerned. However, if you experience hefty bleeding, are bleeding longer than seven days, consistent bleeding between periods, or your periods are occurring less than twenty-one days apart, you should seek medical attention. You could have underlying issues that need attention.

Chapter Summary

Women experience irregular periods for many reasons: pregnancy, medical conditions, weight gain or loss, breastfeeding, hormonal imbalances, stress, or excessive exercise.

If you are experiencing irregular periods, and you have recently been sexually active, you should take a pregnancy test. If you have recently given birth and are breastfeeding, you will likely experience irregular periods for the duration of your breastfeeding. Other reasons for irregular periods might include certain medications and medical conditions.

On a similar topic, women might also experience metrorrhagia, or bleeding and or spotting between periods. Many women find that using hormonal contraceptive can be useful to regular irregular periods and spotting between menstrual cycles. If you have ruled out most of the causes of irregular periods or spotting and are also experiencing abnormal vaginal discharge, then you should consult with your doctor. This is vital to make sure that you don't have any STIs or other types of infection.

There are also many reasons why a women's period might stop, including pregnancy, breastfeeding, and the menopause. There are also certain medications and medical conditions that can cause amenorrhea, as well as congenital disabilities.

You might be perimenopausal if you experience any symptoms including irregular periods, hot flashes, sleep issues, mood changes, vaginal or bladder problems, decreased fertility, changes in sexual function, loss of bone mass, or changes in cholesterol levels.

The perimenopause can last anywhere between two and ten years. If your perimenopausal symptoms are interfering with your everyday life, then you should seek out assistance from a medical professional to get some relief from your symptoms.

In the next chapter, we are going to discuss the effects that birth control can have on the menstrual cycle.

CHAPTER SEVEN – HOW DOES BIRTH CONTROL INTERFERE WITH MY MENSTRUAL CYCLE?

Ah, birth control — a medical miracle that empowers women to separate sex from procreation. For millennia, men and women had been coming up with unique and sometimes barbaric ways to enjoy sex without having to worry about making a baby; from drinking mercury to shoving crocodile poop up the vagina, birth control has come a long way!

In this chapter, we are going to look at how your menstrual cycle affects your sex drive and why you seem to want sex more or less at different points in your cycle. Then we will move on to the purpose of specific birth control methods and how these birth control methods affect ovulation. We look at why you still need to bleed each month and the side effects of birth control on your body. Finally, we will consider what happens to your body when you stop using birth control.

The Menstrual Cycle and Your Sex Drive

The female libido is a bit of a mystery.

It's common for women to experience a peak in their sex drive during their high and peak ovulation times. There is a distinct, biological reason for this. When a woman is ovulating, their bodies are preparing to become pregnant. While we may not technically go "in heat" as most mammals would, there are times during our cycle that we become more eager for sex. Although unlike mammals, we can become pregnant year-round and are receptive to sexual intercourse any time of the year (Castleman, 2015).

As women, we tend to peak in sexual motivation when we are ovulating. This peak is simply due to biology. During ovulation, our bodies are primed for conception and reproduction, which increases our libido to signal that we are open to making a baby. While this is not the case for most women every month, it did serve as an essential aspect of our biology during the dark ages.

Many researchers have tried to study the link between just ovulation and arousal. However, they found that there is generally a high level of stability between arousal at all points of the menstrual cycle (Castleman, 2015).

In addition to our biological urges to make babies while we are ovulating, many women can be "turned off" from sex before or after their period. This could be due to symptoms of PMS or other discomforts they experienced from their cycle. While sex can help with PMS cramping and other symptoms, many women usually don't feel hot when they feel like throwing up or are having a headache.

Ovulation can undoubtedly play a role in how willing a woman is for sex during her cycle, but it is not the sole factor. Other factors include hormonal birth control, work, and relationship status. The pill is a hormonal contraceptive which alters the natural menstrual cycle which can, in turn, alter a woman's libido. However, women who do not take a hormonal contraceptive will still experience changes in their monthly sexual desire (Castleman, 2015). Women who experience a lot of stress at work have a decrease in their libido and a decreased interest in sex.

However, the same women who experience a decrease in sexual desire during the workweek can experience an uptake in sexual interest while on vacation and away from their stress stimulus. Lastly, there is a stark difference in sex between women who are in long-term, committed relationships and those who are single. Most notably, single women tend to have a spike in libido during ovulation, while those in long-term relationships generally do not (Castleman, 2015).

If you feel you have decreases and spikes in your feelings around sex, you should journal that as well. It might be beneficial to plan date nights and romantic getaways around the times you are feeling more sexual. Don't be afraid to communicate these things your partner either. It's not common for male partners to follow their female partner's menstrual cycle to determine when they should make sexual advances. However, having an honest conversation can help with your sexual relationship. You can start a journal about your desires during certain times of your cycle, and share it with your partner, so they can better understand how you are feeling. Talking about this directly to your partner can be uncomfortable; however, writing things down to share with them is an effective and efficient way to communicate and strengthen your relationship.

Fun Fact: Women who have a higher *soy* diet tend to have a *lower* libido - just one more reason to watch what you are eating (depending on your goals, *wink-wink*).

The hormones responsible for sexual desire in women are estrogen and **testosterone**.

Yes, contrary to popular belief, testosterone is also present in women.

Testosterone is associated with sexual desire in both men and women. Women produce testosterone in both the ovaries and adrenal glands (men in the testes), although only about one-tenth of what men generally produce (MacLeod, 2018).

Many factors come into play to determine if we are sexually (and mentally) available for our partner. Don't beat yourself up if you're not feeling in the mood. You may have things on your mind, or you have been stressing out over something. It's best to try to talk things over with your partner instead of keeping your stress inside.

The Purpose of Various Birth Control Methods

There are roughly eighteen different kinds of birth control, ranging from the pill to abstinence. The types that we are going to cover in a little more in-depth are hormonal birth controls. These are the kind of birth control that will interfere with your hormones and possibly your menstrual cycle.

The different types of hormonal birth control include implants (in your arm), IUDs, shots, vaginal rings, patches, and the pill. Other forms of birth control, such as male and female condoms, diaphragms, sponges, cervical caps, spermicides all prevent pregnancy and or the transmission of STIs via spermicides and barriers. These forms of contraception do not contain hormones and should not have any effect on your menstrual cycle. Various types of birth control, such as fertility awareness, breastfeeding, abstinence, tubal ligation, and vasectomies, can also mess with your menstrual cycle but do not introduce synthetic hormones.

We're going to look at hormonal birth control methods, the purpose of each, and how they can each affect your menstrual cycle.

Contraceptive Implant

The **contraceptive implant** is a small rod about the size of a matchstick. An implant is an excellent option for women who are looking for a "set it and forget it" type of birth control. A doctor places it under the skin of your upper arm, and it can help prevent pregnancy for up to five years. It releases progestin, which helps to prevent sperm from reaching the egg and fertilizing it; it does this by thickening the mucus in the cervix. **Progestin** also helps to prevent ovulation, and no egg means no pregnancy (Planned Parenthood, 2019). This prevention of ovulation can also cause changes in your menstrual cycle.

An implant is an excellent option for younger women or even teenagers. It doesn't release a lot of hormones, and they won't have to worry about forgetting to take the pill. If a woman decides later in life that she would like to have a baby, the implant can be easily removed for regular ovulation to resume.

The initial installation may cause some bruising and soreness at the site. However, any bruising or discomfort is only temporary. Either your general practitioner or a trained nurse can perform the procedure right in their office with a local anaesthetic. Some women might also experience amenorrhea as a side effect of the implant (NHS, 2019).

You should not use a contraceptive implant if you have a history of blood clots, liver disease, uterine cancer, or are already experiencing unusual vaginal bleeding. Make sure you speak with your doctor before you get the implant and let them know if you experience high blood pressure, diabetes, depression, high cholesterol, or are overweight. These could lead to potentially harmful side effects (Drugs.com, 2019).

Certain supplements and medications can also have adverse side effects if taken while having a contraceptive implant. If you are taking drugs such as bosentan, griseofulvin, rifampin, St. John's wort, topiramate, any barbiturate, seizure medications, or medications for AIDS or HIV, then you should not get the implant (Drugs.com, 2019). However, this is not a complete list; there are over 170 different drug reactions when using the implant, so make sure you are honest with your doctor and let them know everything you take.

The implant is *99% effective.*

Intrauterine Device

The **intrauterine device**, or **IUD**, is another low-maintenance birth control that is inserted directly into the uterus. The IUD is one of the most effective birth controls out there. It is closest to the uterus, has a high success rate and also delivers the lowest amount of hormones. It's a small, flexible piece of plastic shaped like a T, and there are several kinds available on the market. Hormonal IUDs include Mirena, Kyleena, Liletta, and Skyla. Also, there is a copper IUD which does not contain any hormones called Paragard, which lasts for about twelve years.

Like the birth control arm implant, the hormonal

IUDs release progestin to prevent pregnancy. The Mirena and Liletta brands can prevent pregnancy for up to seven years, while the Kyleena brand can prevent pregnancy for up to five years. The Skyla brand is a little smaller than the other brands but is made for women with smaller uteruses, like women who've yet to have any children. Skyla can prevent pregnancy for up to three years (Planned Parenthood, 2019).

Hormonal IUDs prevent pregnancy the same way the contraceptive implant does. Hormonal IUDs work by thickening the mucus in the cervix to prevent ovulation. Copper IUDs effectively repel sperm, as sperm are not big fans of copper. Same as with the implant, if you decide you want to have a baby, your doctor can easily remove the IUD, and you will be available for baby-making business.

Do not use an IUD if you think you might already be pregnant, have an untreated sexually transmitted infection, have any issues with your pelvis or womb, or experience unexplained bleeding between your periods or after sex (NHS, 2019).

There are also several risks when considering using an IUD. There is a slight chance that you could develop a pelvic infection within the first few weeks of the implant being in place. While it is not very common, your body could reject the IUD, and the womb could expel it or move it out of place. Your doctor or nurse can show you how to check if it's still in place. There is also the potential of causing damage to the womb, which often does not present symptoms. You are also at an increased risk of ectopic pregnancy if the IUD fails to prevent pregnancy. (NHS, 2019).

The IUD, like the implant, is *99% effective*.

Contraceptive Injection Shot

The **contraceptive injection shot** more formally known as the **Depo-Provera shot** is a hormonal injection that you would receive every three months to prevent pregnancy. As with the other forms of hormonal birth control, it contains progestin to thicken the cervical mucus and halt ovulation. A healthcare professional would usually administer the shot; however, you can also apply them yourself if you are receiving the shots from a reliable healthcare centre. The shot is needed every twelve to thirteen weeks, or about four times per year.

Like other forms of birth control, when you first start on the shot, you should add an extra layer of protection like a condom to prevent pregnancy. Furthermore, these birth control methods will NOT stop the transmission of STIs. In all cases, you should be using a condom to avoid contracting STIs.

Some of the hormonal changes that can occur when using the contraceptive injection are irregular periods or increased spotting and breakthrough bleeding. Women might also experience a change in appetite, weight gain, nausea, tender breasts, headaches, and a change in sexual drive and interest (Carter, 2017).

You should not consider using the contraceptive injection if you think you might be pregnant, are worried about a change in menstruation, or are considering having a baby within the next year. You should also avoid the injection if you have a history of heart disease, stroke, liver disease, breast cancer, or are at risk for osteoporosis (NHS, 2019).

Certain medications and supplements can interfere with the contraceptive injection: some seizure medications, certain antibiotics, HIV and AIDS medications, as well as St. John's wort (Vergnaud, 2019).

The birth control shot is *94% effective.*

Vaginal Ring

The **vaginal ring**, otherwise known as the **NuvaRing**, is a safe and effective method of birth control if used correctly. The technique consists of a small, flexible ring that is worn inside the vagina for three weeks and then removed for one week, with a new replacement at the end of the one-week break. It functions by releasing hormones which stop the egg from being fertilized. The hormones estrogen and progestin are absorbed in the body through the vaginal lining and into the bloodstream. The vaginal ring works the same as other hormonal birth control by stopping ovulation and thickening the mucus in your cervix.

There are more than 380 medications and supplements that can cause issues with the vaginal ring. Be extra thorough when describing your medicines to the doctor. Some of the more common drugs that can cause problems include adderall, clonazepam, cymbalta, gabapentin, ibuprofen, lexapro, monistat, and lamictal. (Drugs.com, 2019).

The birth control ring is *91% effective.*

Contraceptive Patch

The contraceptive patch is somewhat like a nicotine patch, but you would wear it on your skin on the area of your belly, butt, upper arm, or back. The patch is placed on the skin for three weeks and then taken off for a week to have your period. Much like the other forms of hormonal birth control, the patch releases estrogen and progestin directly through the skin.

Some women may not experience any adverse side effects of using the contraceptive patch. However, others may experience some potentially severe side effects similar to PMS symptoms. These side effects can include bleeding or spotting between periods, fatigue, fluid retention, skin irritations, mood swings, muscle cramps or spasms, nausea, vaginal discharge, or vomiting. If you are experiencing any of these side effects, you should contact your doctor and investigate other forms of birth control (Ernst, 2018).

Many women find it beneficial to place the patch in different areas upon each use to reduce potential irritation. Despite this strategy, do not place the patch on skin that's already sore or irritated, like areas with eczema or psoriasis. It should also not be placed on areas where it could be rubbed off by tight clothing. Lastly, do not place the patch on your breasts.

You should not use the patch if you think you are pregnant or are breastfeeding a baby that is less than six weeks old. It is also not advised to use the contraceptive patch if you are over the age of thirty-five and smoke or have quit smoking in the past twelve months. You should also avoid using the patch if you have lupus, breast cancer, diabetes, blood clots, high blood pressure, or migraines. It's ill-advised as well to use the contraceptive patch if you are overweight or are taking certain medications or supplements (NHS, 2019).

Medications for AIDS and HIV, epilepsy, tuberculosis antibiotics, St. John's wort and general antibiotics should be avoided when using the patch for contraception (NHS, 2109).

The birth control patch is *91% effective* when used correctly.

Combined Oral Contraceptive Pill

Probably the most well-known of hormonal birth controls is the oral contraceptive pill. Whereas the other methods of hormonal birth control last for weeks or even years, the birth control pill needs to be taken daily to be effective. Like all other forms of hormonal birth control, the birth control pill prevents pregnancy by inhibiting fertilization, stopping ovulation, and thickening the mucus in the cervix.

Many birth control pills adhere to the twenty-eight day cycle, and some can prevent menstruation for up to three months at a time. These contraceptives contain twenty-one days of active hormone contraceptive pills followed by seven days of sugar (placebo) pills, during which menstruation would take place (Mayo Clinic Staff, 2017).

Many women often opt for using the pill to help with heavy periods or painful PMS symptoms. Minor side effects of taking the pill can include mood swings, nausea, breast tenderness, and headaches. While some claim weight gain as a side effect, there is no known evidence of this. Women have also reported a change in sexual desire when taking the pill, as well as spotting and irregular bleeding (Planned Parenthood, 2019).

As with all types of contraception, there is the possibility of adverse side effects. Some women might experience vomiting and diarrhoea as a side effect of taking the oral contraceptive pill. As previously mentioned, if you are experiencing any adverse side effects, you should journal them and bring it up with your doctor at your next visit.

There are also many medications that you should avoid while taking the birth control pill. These include but are not limited to carbamazepine, felbamate, oxcarbazepine, phenobarbital, phenytoin, primidone, and topiramate. Make sure to consult with your general practitioner if you are taking any of these medications and are planning on taking the combined contraceptive pill.

When the pill is used properly, it is *91% effective*. However, this percentage goes down every time a woman forgets to take the pill or doesn't refill her prescription on time. Conversely, it rises the more faithful a woman is taking the pill (meaning by the minute, every day). I found it useful to set a reminder on either my phone or a physical alarm clock. This helped me to remember to take the pill consistently at the correct time each day. If you ever are late taking your pill, or have forgotten to take your pill completely, be extra careful when engaging in sexual intercourse. Always use a condom to prevent unwanted pregnancies and the transmission of STIs.

Birth Control and Ovulation: Why You Need to Bleed Every Month

If there is one thing that many of the hormonal birth controls have in common is that they stop ovulation from occurring. Some varieties of birth control also help and control metrorrhagia, or if you remember, breakthrough bleeding, which is bleeding or spotting between your menstrual cycle or during pregnancy

(Sullivan, 2018).

Breakthrough bleeding can have many different factors such as switching birth control, contracting an STD, or having an inflammatory condition or a sensitive cervix. It can also occur if you are experiencing an ectopic pregnancy or miscarriage, fibroids, or hematoma during pregnancy.

Many contraceptives can cause breakthrough bleeding when you are beginning a new birth control regime. Even if you are taking your pill every day on the dot, you might still experience breakthrough bleeding. This occurs as the combination of progesterone and estrogen prevent ovulation from occurring while also changing the consistency of the cervical mucus (Pandia Health, 2019).

When you first start taking birth control pills, or any other type of hormonal birth control, it can take some time for your body to adjust. During this adjustment period, you may experience breakthrough bleeding. You may also experience inconsistent bleeding if you change the time of day that you take the pill, or if you miss a pill.

If you continue to experience irregular bleeding, you should contact your doctor.

Birth control that is most likely to cause breakthrough bleeding include:

- Monthly birth control pills or patches.
- Any birth control that contains ethinyl estradiol and levonorgestrel that assist in prolonging the time between periods.
- IUDs that are both hormonal and copper within the first three months of being implanted into the cervix.
- The Depo shot.
- Vaginal rings.

If you are experiencing bleeding between periods while taking any of these forms of birth control, you should consult with your general practitioner. Typically, breakthrough bleeding is not a concern when taking hormonal birth control. You should only be concerned if you are also experiencing pain, if bleeding is frequently happening, or it is abnormally heavy (Pandia Health, 2019).

Breakthrough bleeding can usually last anywhere from eight to twelve weeks when you switch birth control. If the bleeding persists after the twelve weeks, you should consult your doctor. At this point, your doctor might prescribe estrogen to regulate your period.

If you have been taking hormonal birth control pills for an extended time, this can also cause breakthrough bleeding. Many doctors recommend taking a break from hormonal birth control for extended periods to avoid potential health complications. Taking the pill can potentially cause blood clotting, which can lead to more health problems such as stroke, deep vein thrombosis (DVT), and pulmonary embolism (Tantry, 2019).

What Are the Side Effects of Birth Control on Your Body?

Whenever you introduce any external substance into your body, there are going to be side effects. Many women believe taking hormonal contraceptives just help to prevent pregnancy. However, while taking an oral contraceptive can be very effective against preventing pregnancy, it can also offer additional benefits and side effects. Some of the benefits of taking an oral contraceptive include relief from menstrual and PMS pain as well as an improved skin condition.

Almost all the hormonal contraceptives prevent pregnancy in a similar fashion, from preventing ovulation, thickening the mucus in the cervix to avoid fertilization, and stopping ovulation. (Ernst, 2018).

Side effects of taking hormonal birth control include:

- Lack of protection against STIs.
- Loss of, decrease, or excessive bleeding during menstruation; spotting or bleeding between periods.
- Vaginal irritation.
- Breast enlargement and or tenderness.
- Changes in sex drive.

Besides, taking hormonal birth control can slightly increase your risk of cervical cancer. Researchers question if the increased risk of cervical cancer is due to an increased risk of HPV or the use of hormonal birth control (Ernst, 2018).

Some women who also experience migraines find that taking hormonal contraceptives make them worse; the estrogen tends to aggravate the migraines.

If you want to decrease any severe side effects from taking oral contraceptives, being smoke-free is a great start. It's been shown that women who smoke tend to experience more severe side effects from taking oral and hormonal birth control. Two significant side effects are an increase in blood pressure, in addition to a higher risk of developing blood clots.

These health risks become even higher if you are over the age of thirty-five and smoke, experience high blood pressure, or have any pre-existing heart conditions or diabetes. Many women can use hormonal birth control without experiencing any side effects, but some women do experience side effects that are potentially serious (Ernst, 2018). These side effects are why you require a prescription and routine monitoring from a general practitioner for hormonal birth control. If at any point when you are taking hormonal birth control, you feel pain in your chest, are coughing up blood, or feel faint, you should contact your doctor immediately.

Although many side effects of taking hormonal birth control are physical, numerous women experience psychological changes as well. It's not uncommon for women taking hormonal contraceptives to undergo more severe mood swings and depression (Ernst, 2018). Our bodies try to maintain homeostasis by keeping our hormones balanced. Often when we introduce synthetic hormones into our bodies, it disrupts our homeostasis. This disturbance can result in changes in our mood, specifically the addition of depression.

It's uncommon for women taking hormonal contraceptives to experience changes in their weight and appetite, although it may happen. If you are looking to avoid weight gain or changes in your appetite when taking an oral contraceptive, a progestin-only contraceptive is advised. Remember to always consult with your general practitioner to determine what type of contraception is best of you personally.

While it might be convenient to blame birth control for changes in weight directly, it is natural for hormones to play a part in regulating our eating habits. If you are experiencing weight gain, refer to your journal. This action will help to determine if there have been any lifestyle changes that you have made that may be affecting your weight.

Some women may also experience symptoms similar to PMS, such as nausea and bloating when taking hormonal contraceptives (HealthLine, 2018). However, these symptoms tend to subside after a few weeks, when your body has become used to the extra hormones.

It can be tricky to predict how a woman's body will respond to hormonal contraceptives. Some women experience adverse side effects such as an increase in unwanted hair growth, while others experience positive side effects such as an improvement in acne-prone skin, overall skin tone and a decrease in unwanted hair growth. There tends to be some degree of trial and error when determining birth control options with your doctor (Ernst, 2018).

What Happens When You Stop Using Birth Control?

If you decide to cease your usage of hormonal birth control, there is the possibility that you will experience some side effects or other symptoms. Unlike antidepressants or antipsychotics, there is no prescribed method for when you decide to stop using hormonal birth control after a long period of use. Generally, if you are taking an oral contraceptive, whenever in the pack that you stop taking it, you will likely have your period immediately afterwards. Some women who have accidentally skipped multiple pills consecutively will notice this change event as well (Shkodzik, 2019). Not every woman will necessarily experience this; some may take longer to adjust to the hormonal changes.

Some of the more common side effects that occur when you stop taking hormonal birth control are:

- Inconsistent, irregular, heavier, or painful periods; spotting.
- Acne.
- Mood swings.
- Weight loss or weight gain.

Often, women experience erratic or irregular periods after stopping hormonal birth control. It takes time for your body to adjust to the new, natural hormone levels.

This is like the withdrawal of any other type of drug. Depending on the type of hormonal birth control you were using, it could take up to a full year for your periods to regulate.

Considering hormonal birth control pills contain estrogen, many women experience weight loss after they stop taking it. This effect is due to a reduction in fluid retention that estrogen causes. It's less common for women to *gain* weight after they stop taking birth control; however, it's still possible. If you experience weight gain upon terminating hormonal birth control, this can easily be remedied by a healthier diet and exercise (Shkodzik, 2019).

Spotting or bleeding in between your periods is possible after you stop taking birth control in the middle of your menstrual cycle. This bleeding is only temporary until your natural hormone levels level out.

Many women, particularly younger women, start using oral contraceptives to minimize cramping and PMS symptoms. Upon terminating oral contraception mid-cycle, some women may experience more intense cramping. If you experience more cramping than usual, you can try some self-care methods like walking or using a heating pad.

The type of hormonal birth control you're using will change when you start ovulating again. For many women who have used the pill, ovulation tends to begin again after just a few weeks. If you were using the birth control shot, it could take much longer for ovulation to resume (Shkodzik, 2019). If you are trying to conceive and have recently come off birth control, you should start tracking your cycle to determine when your high and peak ovulation days are. You can track your cycle by taking your basal body temperature daily, examining your vaginal discharge, or using a home ovulation test.

Chapter Summary

It's natural for women to experience a peak in sexual desire while ovulating, which is a biological side effect of procreation. Unlike other mammals that only go into heat a few times per year, women can become pregnant and desire sex year-round.

Other factors that can contribute to sexual desire

include the use of hormonal birth control, work stress, and relationship status. The use of hormonal birth control can cause an increase or decrease in sexual desire. Stress from work might put a strain on a woman's desires, and her libido could also diminish the longer she is in a committed relationship.

The ups and downs you experience in your sexual desires are entirely normal. There are some things you can journal about and share with your doctor or partner. Open communication is essential for a healthy relationship.

The use of hormonal birth control methods can also play a significant role in your menstrual cycle and how you feel. Forms such as the implant, IUD, and shot all halt ovulation, making them effective at preventing pregnancy; however, they can also cause irregular menstruation.

Introducing foreign chemicals into your body is always going to have some side effects, specifically with hormonal birth control. The use of hormonal birth control can lead to spotting or bleeding between periods, vaginal irritation, changes in libido, breast enlargement and tenderness, and loss of, decrease, or excessive bleeding during menstruation. You can reduce your risk of side effects by making lifestyle changes like not smoking or drinking in excess and maintaining a healthy body weight and diet.

You can also experience symptoms when you stop using birth control. These symptoms include spotting, inconsistent and irregular periods, skin issues, mood swings, heavy and painful periods, and weight gain or weight loss.

Many women choose to start taking hormonal birth control to minimize symptoms of PMS and to regulate their periods.

In the next chapter, we will go over self-care strategies and the best ways to feel comfortable while on your period.

CHAPTER EIGHT – HOW TO FEEL COMFORTABLE DURING YOUR PERIOD: A SELF-CARE GUIDE

Self-care is vital for everybody. It is just as important to take care of ourselves, as it is to care about other people. Self-care looks different for every woman. For some, it is a glass of wine and a good book by the fire; for others, it's a nice walk in the park or shopping centre with friends. When it comes to your period, there are many ways in which you can care for yourself.

In this chapter, we will focus on sanitation products, how to use them and the pros and cons of each one. We will discuss period poverty and how to maximize your comfort while travelling, working, or going to school or college. Finally, we will talk about how changing your lifestyle can impact your periods.

Types of Sanitation Products

There are two main types of female sanitation products: internal and external. Internal products include tampons and menstrual disks, and external products include pads and panty liners. Internal products are inserted into the body to catch the flow of menstrual blood, whereas external products are worn on the outside of the body to line the underwear to catch menstrual blood.

<u>Fun Fact:</u> Some of the first tampons were small pieces of wood wrapped with lint… *Ouch!*

The FDA in the US and the MHRA in the UK approve external and internal feminine hygiene products before they are released to ensure safety. While the risk is quite low, using tampons puts you at risk for **toxic shock syndrome (TSS)**. TSS is rare, but it can be fatal. TSS is caused when Staphylococcus aureus (staph bacteria) overgrow in the body, due to leaving in a tampon for too long, which then releases toxins into the body. TSS is most commonly linked to the use of super-absorbent tampons, and it is still possible to contract TSS when using diaphragms, cervical caps, and menstrual sponges (Todd, 2001). TSS can be avoided by changing your tampon or feminine hygiene product every few hours.

If you experience any of the following symptoms, you should contact your doctor immediately as they may mean signs and symptoms of TSS:

- Confusion or dizziness.
- Seizures.
- Intense headaches.
- Muscle aches (not related to exercise).
- Vomiting or diarrhoea.
- Low blood pressure.
- Sudden fever; rash on palms or soles of the feet that look like a sunburn.

Symptoms of TSS appear quickly and can cause trauma, renal failure, and even death (Mayo Clinic Staff, 2017).

There are many kinds of period products on the market today. Although their respective federal departments may have approved them, many feminine hygiene products still contain chemicals and synthetic ingredients (CYWH, 2018). Women are becoming more and more mindful about handling their periods in a natural way. This action has led to a rise in more natural feminine hygiene products.

Period Panties

Period panties are like pads but are an entire pair of underwear rather than just a lining. They are the newest form of female hygiene product on the market and have been well taken to by the people who've used them. The crotch of the panties is four layers thick and can be worn with or without additional protection (CYWH, 2018). They are made for use with light and reasonable period flow and are both reusable and washable.

They can be a little more expensive in the beginning; however, there are some advantages. If washed according to directions, they can last you quite a long time, which in turn will save you a significant amount of money on disposable period products. They are also better for the environment and reduce landfill waste. Nonetheless, these reusable panties are not made to be worn on their own when experiencing heavy periods. This means if you experience a heavy period, you will have to use a disposable option in addition to period panties.

Reusable Cloth Pads

There are reusable diapers, so why not also reusable cloth pads?

The **reusable cloth pads** are like reusable underwear in that you wash them after use. Then you would use them just as you would a regular disposable pad. They are made up of two parts: the liner and the liner holder. The liner holder has wings that snap to each other to secure the pad to your underwear. The liner itself is then placed inside of the liner holder and is taken out to be washed after use. These tend to be a little more affordable than reusable panties and help prevent adding to landfills. These are also great for girls who are sensitive to chemicals in conventional cotton pads and don't want to use tampons (CYWH, 2018).

All-cotton and Non-chlorine Bleached Pads and Tampons

Did you know that most cotton pads and tampons are bleached and contain pesticides and other chemicals?

Think about that.

If you don't want or can't have these chemicals near your genitals, you're in luck — there exists a 100% organic cotton alternative to pads and tampons. While these can be a little more expensive and still wind up in a landfill, you're at least not exposing yourself to any potentially harmful chemicals (CYWH, 2018).

Sea Sponge Tampons

As it would turn out, some ancient methods of feminine hygiene are still alive and well today, such as using sea sponges to catch menstrual blood. They work the same as regular cotton tampons but are reusable. **Sea sponges** are absorbent, completely natural, contain natural antibacterial properties, and can last up to six months or even longer if properly taken care of (CYWH, 2018).

Like traditional tampons, they have a string attached for easy removal, and you can find various sizes to accommodate the flow of your period. Sea sponge tampons are extremely easy to use and environmentally friendly, not to mention easy to clean and reuse.

The only downside to sea sponge tampons is that they don't come with an applicator for insertion. Nevertheless, once you use them a few times, they are easy enough to insert without an applicator.

Reusable Menstrual Cups

Reusable cups are made of soft silicone or rubber and are inserted into the vagina to catch the menstrual blood. The cup is folded together and easily fits into the vagina without experiencing any discomfort. The cup is usually fitted to the person and can be straightforward enough to insert and remove when it needs to be emptied. All you need to do is remove the cup while sitting over the toilet, rinse out, and reinsert if necessary.

One significant advantage of using a menstrual cup is that they are not linked to TSS, as they merely collect the blood rather than absorb it. Unlike other feminine hygiene products, a menstrual cup can be worn for six to twelve hours. This timeframe, of course, is dependent on how heavy your flow is.

There are two main types of reusable menstrual cups. There is a smaller size for women who have not delivered a baby, and a larger size for women who have given birth vaginally. There is another version of the reusable menstrual cup that can be used during sex.

Pads and Tampons

These are your standard methods of hygiene during menstruation. The most significant advantage of using **pads and tampons** is that they are cheap and easy to come by. Many women often carry extras with them, and they can be found in most general stores and even in vending machines.

There are several disadvantages to using conventional pads and tampons. As I said previously, traditional pads and tampons contain residue of bleach, pesticides, and other chemicals. Any woman can be sensitive to the chemicals used in making conventional pads and tampons. Furthermore, they contribute to a more extensive environmental problem of adding to our increasing landfills.

Period Poverty

I want to share with you a little scenario. You are a homeless woman, already living each day not knowing how you will come by your next hot meal. Your period is irregular due to the stress of your lifestyle and the lack of hormonal birth control to help regulate it. Each time you get your period, you have to determine if you are going to try and steal a pack of pads or tampons from the store, try to break into a tampon vending machine, or steal to stock up just enough money to buy a box of feminine hygiene products.

Or...

You are a young girl living in Nepal. Even though the practice is illegal, your family still uses menstruation huts. It is a small, cold, and damp lodging made of mud and sticks where you have to live for the duration of your period. You are deprived of clean and running water and forced to live in deplorable and unsanitary conditions. This is because your family's culture views you as unclean when you are menstruating. You are not even allowed to touch your loved ones, cattle, green vegetables, or any plants for fear of repercussions from the Gods. Furthermore, you are at risk of dying yourself due to poor healthcare, smoke inhalation (from a fire you're using to try and keep warm) or being attacked by an animal (Gupta & Pokharel, 2019).

What many women might not be aware of is the suffering that some women must endure due to **period poverty.** They may lack access to proper feminine hygiene, or even the basic knowledge of menstruation. This scenario does not only occur with women in poverty in the US and the UK but also other countries. It's a phenomenon that many don't even realize is happening because it is not directly happening to them. We, as people of all genders and ethnicities, need to work together to bring menstrual equality to the world.

Over 800 million women are menstruating on any given day. Women and young girls all over the world are shunned or banished while experiencing menstruation. Specifically, in the US and the UK, period poverty refers more to women being unable to afford proper sanitation products. When young girls don't have access to adequate sanitation products, they miss school, which leads to even further socio-economic issues in the future (Sharma, 2019).

The UK has the right idea with putting an end to period poverty and ensuring that all schools across England have free sanitation products (Sharma, 2019). This plan will help the nearly 12% of girls who miss class due to having their periods and not having access to proper sanitation products. While the UK has taken up the reigns in ensuring girls and women in low-income housing have access to sufficient feminine hygiene products, the US is still behind the times.

With nearly 14% of girls and women living below the poverty line, there is a huge disparity in access to proper sanitation products. It's not just about having access to pads and tampons. Period poverty often reinforces the poverty cycle, as girls and women must resort to archaic measures to care for themselves. It is embarrassing enough to have to walk around with wads of toilet paper in your underwear. On top of this, girls and women that experience period poverty can experience the same kinds of pain and discomfort as those who have access to proper sanitation products (Sharma, 2019).

Although the US means well by implementing a bill that forces schools, correctional facilities, and homeless shelters to provide sanitation products, it is in vain. The facilities themselves bear the costs of funding this initiative. Schools are suffering the most significant need, but sanitation dispensers can cost upwards of $8,000 (Sharma, 2019). While it's a sad fact, pads and tampons are still labelled as "luxury items."

Local governments could easily fund the bill to provide proper female sanitation products as it should be within the state's budget. Items like band-aids, soap, condoms, sunscreen, and toilet paper are all readily available.

Not only are pads and tampons not free to those in need, but many are also still taxed on them. In the US, women and girls pay a "tampon tax" that can add up to over $800 in a woman's lifetime of menstruation (Cora, 2019).

Many women already struggle to put food on the table and keep a roof over their heads, so the average $7 per month for sanitation products can be too much for some. Many items deemed as necessary, such as groceries and medication, are tax-free while adequate sanitation products are still taxed (Sharma, 2019).

Three main things perpetuate period poverty within the US: the stigma of discussions around menstruation, financial hardship, and lack of access to proper sanitation products. The lack of access to products also possesses an increased health risk of TSS when women try to wear tampons longer than they should so they can save some money (Sharma, 2019).

Unfortunately, talking about periods and the menstrual cycle is still taboo. However, we are making some progress here and there. So, keep these points in mind when you go to the store to buy your next pack of tampons. It's good to be consciously aware of all these situations.

How to Maximize Your Comfort When Travelling, Working, or Going to School

Having your period is never fun, especially if you suffer from PMS symptoms. Whether you are travelling, going to work, or attending school, having your period can make your day a little less enjoyable. There are things you can do to make your day suck a little less.

One of these strategies is always to be *prepared.*

It doesn't matter if you are flying off to Bali, working a double shift, or pulling an all-nighter for a big exam. You should always make sure that you are prepared and have a period emergency kit nearby. The kit should include sanitation products, wet wipes, pain killers, an extra pair of panties, and anything else you deem necessary. Even if you are expertly tracking your period, you never know what can happen. This is especially true if you are traveling, you never know when you will have access to purchase pads or tampons if the need were to arise (WomanLog, 2019).

Don't forget about sexual protection, as well. If you are travelling, working, or studying long hours, make sure that you are keeping up with your birth control if applicable. You should also consider protection during sex too to prevent STIs.

Especially if you are travelling, you should take the weather and your activities into consideration. You should already be conscious of the details of your period, such as if certain days are worse than others. It's useful to think about it when you're planning your itinerary. It helps to try not to do anything strenuous on the days that you are going to feel worse. Also make sure you are drinking plenty of water while on your period, particularly if it's going to be hot outside (WomanLog, 2019). Going from one extreme weather condition to another can potentially mess with your cycle. Therefore, you should make sure that you are always going into your adventures prepared.

Part of being prepared includes effectively tracking your period via a good journal or period tracking app. Tracking your period can help you to anticipate and plan for work, school, or vacation. You should aim to include when you get your period, how long it lasts, and how heavy your flow is. Also include changes in your vaginal discharge, as well as side effects, before, during, and after your period (Tampax, 2019).

Swimming

If you are comfortable with using a tampon, there is no reason that you shouldn't be able to enjoy the pool or beach while on vacation. If you are not comfortable wearing a tampon, you can wear period underwear or a period swimsuit, which offer extra protection while swimming. Don't forget that if you submerge yourself in water, the water will also help to hold off your period for a while. You can also opt for a very dark or black swimsuit in case you do leak (WomanLog, 2019).

How Lifestyle Changes Can Impact Your Periods

There are many lifestyle changes that you can implement to help reduce period pain and make your life a little easier.

Exercise

In chapter one, I mentioned that exercise could help to relieve menstrual cramping. Even though the thought of heading to the gym sounds like a no go, it offers so many valuable benefits. Working out can help to regulate your hormones, which in all honesty seems like an excellent idea to me!

Hip and Pelvic-opening Exercises

Try to incorporate some stretching exercises or some yoga into your self-care routine to help relieve your PMS symptoms. When I was having a lot of difficulty with my PMS symptoms, I would turn to yoga; I would also suggest it for my patients as well. Yoga not only helps to relieve stress but also to relax your body and your muscles, which can help to ease period pain. Below are some yoga moves that are easy enough for just about anyone to do, even if you aren't flexible, to help you get started. If you feel none of these yoga poses work for you, you can find several functional hip opening exercises by searching "hip opening exercises" online.

Downward Dog

Downward dog is a great exercise to open up the hips and lengthen your spine. To do the pose, begin with your hands on the floor in a table position. Make sure that your wrists are aligned under your shoulders and your knees are directly under your hips. Stretch out your elbows and relax your upper back. Then spread your fingers wide apart and press firmly through your palms, distributing your weight through your hands.

Exhale as you tuck your toes and lift your knees off of off the floor. Then reach your pelvis up towards the ceiling, pointing your butt towards the wall behind you. Begin to straighten your legs but don't lock your knees. At this point, your body should be in the shape of an upside-down V. Keep the pressure evenly distributed through your hands and feet. Hold this position for five to ten breaths, then release by slowly coming back down to the table position.

Crescent Lunge

The crescent lunge can either be done individually or in a series of yoga poses. You can begin in the downward-facing dog position, then step your right foot forward between your hands. Your knee should be bent at a 90-degree angle directly, aligned right above your heel. Your back leg should be straightened out entirely while drawing your hips forward.

Inhale and raise your chest into an upright position while sweeping your arms above your head. Open your palms, so they face one another and tilt your head so that you are looking up towards your hands. Hold this position for up to one to five minutes, then breathe and release, and return to downward-facing dog position.

Pigeon Pose

The pigeon pose is fantastic for opening up your hips, which can help to relieve some of the symptoms associated with PMS. While on all fours, bring your right knee forward toward your wrists, which should be positioned right below your shoulders. This position should stretch your outer hip without any discomfort to your knees. Slide your other leg back and point your toes while keeping your heel pointed towards the ceiling. Slowly press your hips into the floor, hold this position for five to ten breaths.

Lizard Pose

The lizard pose is another yoga pose that can be

done from the downward-facing dog position.

***Tip** - between each post return to downward-facing dog, then transition into the next pose.

Step your right foot forward so that the inside of your foot is facing your pinky finger. Slowly lower your left knee down to the ground. Make sure that your right knee is behind your right foot and that you are not moving too far forward. Your weight should be evenly distributed across both of your hips. Use your weight to sink your hips down. Keep your chin lifted and your chest open.

Hold this position for five to ten breaths then release and return to the downward-facing dog position.

Not only is working out good for you during your period, but it's also beneficial in the long-term. Exercise helps to support your overall physical and mental health and reduce the risk of age-related diseases and conditions. It can help you physically, and it also releases those amazing "feel-good" hormones which serve to ward off things like depression and other mental health disorders.

But what are the best kinds of exercise and what types of exercise should you avoid?

The amount, intensity, and form of exercise you do while on your period will vary drastically. It depends on many factors, such as your PMS symptoms and how heavy your flow is.

Walking is a great way to exercise, especially if you're not used to working out much. You don't need any special equipment and can do it just about anywhere. You can go on short walks and vary your speed depending on how you are feeling.

Light cardio and aerobic exercise are also great. Notice I said "light" — meaning this type of workout should not be as strenuous as, for example, high-intensity interval training (HIIT) workouts. Think of shorter and more comfortable versions of exercises that you would typically do (Klepchukova, 2018). Taking a leisurely bike ride, a few laps in the pool, or even walking up and down steps. Just make sure you're moving.

Strength training is an excellent option for many people. Remember when we covered the menopause that

I said women tend to lose bone mass as they age? Strength training can help to combat that bone loss. You don't have to do a bunch of deadlift squats or max out on the bench press, but some lighter and less intense strength training can help to keep your weight in check as well.

Stretching and balance exercise is great at working on your core muscles while promoting relaxation. Practising Yoga, Pilates, and Tai Chi benefits both your physical and mental health and can aid in relieving stress and tension (Klepchukova, 2018). However, you aren't going to want to try any *inversion poses*.

When exercising on your period, you are going to want to avoid putting additional stress on your body. Therefore, you should avoid super strenuous exercises and inversion poses. Overdoing any strenuous activities while on your period can cause increased inflammation and additional fatigue. Inversion exercises performed in yoga should also be avoided. When you turn upside-down, the ligaments that support the uterus stretch, which could cause damage to the veins and increase bleeding, leading to vascular congestion (Klepchukova,

2018). Also, make sure that you are listening to your body when you are exercising. If you are starting to feel overly exhausted, nauseous, or your pain and discomfort begin to increase to unbearable levels, then you must stop immediately and rest. If these symptoms persist, then you should consult your general practitioner for further investigation.

During a workout while on your period, feminine hygiene is *extra* important. Make sure you're changing your underwear and showering right after you are finished working out. You should also be changing your pad or tampon shortly after working out and putting on fresh clothes as well. If you are concerned about leaking, you can wear both a tampon and a pad or period underwear.

Nutrition

Whether you are on your period or not, you're not going to feel your best chowing down on burgers and bingeing on ice cream. Though there is nothing wrong with a few spoonfuls here and there, it's worth noting that nutrition is still as vital as it always is. Just like your period, nutrition is personal, and what works for one person during their period is not always going to work for another. Some women feel their best when they are eating a strict vegan diet, while others prefer the keto diet. Some like to balance their food between meat and vegetables. You need to be able to figure out what works best for you and makes you feel your best.

Eating regular meals and not going for long periods without eating can help to make you feel better. It can also decrease any associated symptoms of PMS, such as bloating or water retention. While it is okay to have a treat occasionally, make sure that you are mostly eating a healthy and nutritionally balanced diet that makes you feel good. Make sure that you are getting enough healthy fats, protein, and carbs. You should try different ratios of fats, carbs, and proteins to see what works best for you.

Nutrition is not just about making your cramps feel better. It can also help you to control your weight, improve your skin, and keep your energy levels up. If you are someone who struggles with nutrition, you can find additional help by speaking with a nutritionist. Meal planning is always a great idea. Having your meals planned (and keeping junk food to a minimum) will help to curb those impulse behaviours for late-night ice cream binges.

Nutrition can also include things like supplements, hydration, and caffeine consumption. Certain supplements, such as vitamin D and calcium, can ease cramping and other pains associated with menstruation. Many other herbal supplements can help to relieve symptoms associated with PMS and menstruation (Stöppler, 2019).

When you consume a lot of caffeine, you tend to retain more water. Cutting back on your caffeine intake can help to reduce that bloated, crampy, and achy feeling. If you tend to consume a lot of soda, do your best to cut back on it — other healthier alternatives include mineral water and ginger ale. Caffeine is present in more than just coffee; sodas contain a lot of caffeine as well, as does chocolate and tea. Instead of reaching for a giant candy bar when the cravings hit, opt for some quality dark chocolate (Tampax, 2019).

Staying hydrated also has many benefits far beyond

just helping with your period. Drinking enough water will help you to eliminate excess fluid in your body (even though it may seem odd to drink water while feeling bloated). So, make sure to have a water bottle beside you for when you're feeling thirsty. It's not fun to become dehydrated while menstruating (or at any time). If the thought of drinking a gallon of water a day is already daunting, then try flavouring it with fruit or drinking herbal tea.

Recipes to Relieve Menstrual Cramps

There are several great hot drinks out there that you can incorporate into your routine to help reduce some of your menstrual cramps. Here are just a few you can add to your daily routine.

Mint Water

Warm up some water and add either fresh mint leaves or a drop or two of pure mint extract.

Lemon Water

Lemon water is an excellent choice for so many reasons; it helps with clear skin, digestion, and to clear out all the mucus in your chest. You can either drink it at room temperature or in cold water; with lemons soaking in it and a splash of lemon juice and honey.

Broth

Bone broths are beneficial in many ways. They help with collagen production (which means great skin) and are very soothing. Add a dash of sea salt to boost the mineral content.

Teas

Any herbal tea is going to be great for helping to make you feel relaxed and to ease menstrual pain. If you like to sweeten your tea, try using natural sweeteners like honey or stevia instead of sugar.

Get Enough Sleep

Sleeping well is just as important as any other lifestyle adjustment. Teens especially need a couple of extra hours of sleep to feel their best. As an adult, you should get about eight hours of sleep per night; teenagers will need about nine to ten. Try and create a pleasant sleeping environment where you are cool and comfortable and try to lower the number of active stimuli around while you sleep (for example, phones and television). Experts advise for both teens and adults to turn off all electronics for about an hour before bed and do something to help you relax, like reading a book (Gunnars, 2019).

Getting enough good sleep isn't just required during your period; it should be something you practice all the time. Poor sleep can lead to depression, diabetes, and an increase in obesity (Gunnars, 2019). I mentioned before about turning off all electronics around an hour before bed — electronics emit an artificial blue light which can lead to sleep problems.

All light is made up of different coloured wavelengths: blue, red, white, and so on. The sun has a mixture of both of these to help tell your internal clock that it's daytime, and you should wake up. When you look at **blue light** (light emitted from your electronic screens), right before you try to go to sleep, your brain interprets that light as daytime light. This, in turn, causes you to feel less sleepy (Gunnars, 2019).

While it is best to turn off the electronics altogether, you can try wearing blue light blocking glasses. These glasses will help to obstruct the blue light and won't mess with your natural sleep patterns. Sleep masks are also a great option if you need absolute darkness while you sleep.

Other Types of Therapy

Therapy in this context can mean heat therapy, massage therapy, or even CBTs if needed. There are also excellent counselling therapies if you would like to discuss issues related to menstruation, or even life in general.

Heat therapy is good at helping relieve menstrual cramping. Apply a heat wrap or heating pad to your abdomen when you are experiencing period pain. Taking a hot shower or applying a heat patch can work. Heat therapy can help to reduce cramps associated with your period drastically if used in conjunction with over-the-counter painkillers.

Massage therapy can also be beneficial, and who doesn't want another excuse to get a massage. You can use self-massage and gently massage your stomach for a few minutes to help relieve menstrual cramps and increase blood flow. Having a professional massage done can also ease tension and stress, and move your lymphatic system, which will help with draining fluid. Massage, in combination with essential oils such as clary sage, lavender, and marjoram, can also help to ease pain (Stöppler, 2019).

Face masks can also be soothing and beneficial, both for your skin and for stress relief. You can easily make simple face masks at home with ingredients right out of your kitchen.

Avocado Face Mask

Take half of an avocado and mash it up, then rub it all over your skin. The healthy fats will make your skin feel soft and luxurious. To wash off, simply take a warm, wet cloth and place it over your face, then gently wipe the avocado off.

Berries and Yogurt Face Mask

Berries and yoghurt together are great for fighting inflammation in the skin and reducing any puffiness. In a blender, combine two tablespoons of plain yoghurt, two tablespoons of honey, a quarter cup of berries, and one tablespoon of lemon juice. Slather on the skin and leave on for ten to fifteen minutes, then wipe off with a clean damp cloth.

Acupuncture and **acupressure** can also benefit you by reducing PMS symptoms. People are drawn to the ancient Eastern practices of acupuncture and acupressure for their effectiveness. As an added benefit, there are no drugs or medications involved (Stöppler, 2019). While it might be difficult for some women to find access to an acupuncturist, it's worth a try to find relief from symptoms.

Mindfulness meditation is a beautiful practice for relieving stress. It also helps you get better sleep, as it can clear negative feelings that you may be experiencing while on your period. It can also help to manage period pain and even weight loss (Kane, 2018). You can easily incorporate mindful meditation into your everyday life by starting each morning with some reflection. You are also capable of doing it in your car during your lunch break or sitting in your room right before bed. Don't be afraid to try meditating multiple times a day.

To meditate, sit in a quiet area and focus on your breathing. It sometimes helps if you lay on the floor and place your hands on your stomach or chest to help you feel your breath. Before you start, come up with a mantra to say to yourself, something that makes you feel positive and pleasant. Some go with "I am worth it," or "this too shall pass." While you are sitting or lying down, focus on your breathing and repeat the mantra in your mind.

If you are experiencing a lot of pain, you can do the same type of mindful meditation to help with pain relief. While focusing on your breathing, focus on your pain. Allow your body to feel that pain, then let it go.

Chapter Summary

Self-care is so essential for your well-being, whether you are on your period or not. You should find out what works best for you and make sure to work that into your routine. Self-care for you could be having a glass of wine by the fireplace or running a couple of miles at the gym.

Finding the best type of birth control for you might take some trial and error, and the same can be said for sanitation products. Whichever product you choose, make sure you are comfortable with using it. If you decide to use tampons, make sure that you are changing them often as to avoid TSS or any other infections.

Period poverty is alive and well across the world. The UK has taken significant measures to ensure no girls or women must go without adequate protection. However, it seems that the US and many other countries still have a lot of catching up to do.

You can maximize your comfort on your period while travelling, going to school, or working. The best ways to achieve this is always to be prepared, use protection during sex and consider your everyday activities. Some of the lifestyle choices that can impact your period are exercise, sleep, nutrition, and various types of therapies.

PERIODS…JUST WHY?

FINAL WORDS

With all the uncertainty about menstruation and sexuality, it's easy to see why many girls and women are confused about the various functions of their bodies. Having our periods is something that all women have in common, yet there is not nearly enough discussion over anything to do with periods.

So many myths, taboos and stigmas plague the topic of periods that many women suffer in silence. While menstruation can be messy and painful, it is a beautiful and natural process that girls and women should be able to discuss openly.

We all have a responsibility to ensure that conversations about menstruation remain open for young girls. I hope you found this book humorous, insightful, inspiring, and most of all, educational. I wrote this book intending it to be a guide to young girls and women all over the world. The key aim was to help them demystify the physical and psychological aspects of why we continue to have our periods and how hormones work during the menstrual cycle.

If you are anything like I was when I was younger, you probably had questions while reading this book - lots of them.

Once I became a mother, I knew my daughter would have the same questions I did as a young girl. I wanted to be able to equip her with all the answers that she needed about the joys and pains she will experience in womanhood. I wanted my daughter to be confident about her body. I also wanted the same thing for all the girls and women whom I worked with over my forty years as a nurse.

I have gone through having my first period to having my last, and everything in between. I have experienced severe and mild PMS symptoms, light to heavy bleeding, pregnancy, and maybe an accident here and there as well.

I wasn't just looking to educate myself or my daughter. I wanted to be able to spread the word that menstruation is normal, and we should be talking about it openly. I hope that reading this book has brought you the knowledge you need, as well as some fun facts that you can share with your friends. It is a light-hearted way to break the ice when it comes to talking about periods.

You no longer have to agonize, and continually guess each month, as to how you are going to feel when your period shows up. Take your body and your life into your own hands and do what you can to make your period more pleasant. However, don't forget about those who don't have access to proper sanitation products or are living in horrendous conditions because they are menstruating. Try leaving a couple extra pads or tampons in the bathroom at school or work with a sweet little note or give some to a woman or girl in need.

Image Credit: Shutterstock.com

GLOSSARY OF TERMS

Adenomyosis: When womb tissue becomes embedded in the lining of the womb causing heavy bleeding.

Amenorrhea: Abnormal absence of menstruation.

Androgen: Sex hormones that encourage male characteristics to develop in the body (usually testosterone).

Anus: Outermost part of the colon in which waste is expelled.

Asymptomatic: Describing a person who does not show symptoms of a particular condition.

Bacterial Vaginosis: Disease of the vagina that is caused by excessive growth of bacteria.

Cervix: Lower part of the uterus that dilates to accommodate the birth of a baby.

Chlamydia: Sexually transmitted infection caused by parasitic bacteria resulting in discoloured vaginal discharge and other symptoms.

Clitoris: The small, sensitive, erectile part of the female genitals at the anterior end of the vulva.

Cognitive Behavioural Therapy (CBT): Psychotherapy that concentrates on an individual's beliefs and way of thinking to spark a change in their everyday behaviour.

Contraceptive Injection: Injection that prevents pregnancy for about 12 weeks and is 95% effective when used properly.

Contraceptive Implant: Small plastic rod about the size of a matchstick placed into the upper arm and can prevent pregnancy for up to five years, up to 99% effective.

Contraceptive Patch: Patch placed on the skin for three weeks to prevent pregnancy that is up to 91% effective when used properly.

Corpus Luteum: Ruptured follicle during the luteal phase; releases progesterone.

Dopamine: Hormone released during exercise that helps

decrease stress and elevate your mood.

Dysmenorrhea: Painful periods or pain associated with menstruation.

Endometriosis: A condition resulting from the appearance of endometrial tissue outside the uterus and causing pelvic pain.

Endometrium: Membrane made up of mucosal tissue that lines the uterus; helps protect the fetus during pregnancy.

Estrogen: Sex hormones that encourage female characteristics to develop in the body.

Fallopian Tubes: How the egg travels from the ovaries to the uterus.

Fibroids: Benign growth in or around the womb which can lead to heavy or painful periods.

Follicular Phase: Second stage of the menstruation cycle; beginning on the first day of menstruation, the pituitary gland releases follicle-stimulating hormone and immature egg in preparation for fertilization. The uterus also thickens.

Gonadotropin-releasing hormone: A hormone that causes the pituitary gland in the brain to make and secrete the hormones luteinizing hormone (LH) and follicle-stimulating hormone (FSH).

Gonorrhoea: A sexually transmitted infection involving inflammatory discharge from the urethra or vagina.

Hormonal Therapy: Form of treatment that adjusts an individual's hormones (adds, blocks, or removes) to come to a specific result.

Hyperthyroidism: An overactive thyroid gland produces too many hormones, leading to weight loss, irregular heartbeat, and an excessively active metabolism.

Hypothyroidism: An underactive thyroid gland doesn't produce enough hormones, leading to excessive fatigue, weight gain, and depression.

IUD: Intrauterine device; placed directly into the uterus, delivers a low amount of hormones. Shaped like a "T" and made of either plastic or covered in copper, there are several brands and sizes available. IUDs can prevent pregnancy for three to five years, depending on which one you get with up to 99% effectiveness.

Labia majora: Larger outermost folds of the vulva.

Labia Minora: Smaller inner folds of the vulva.

Laparoscopy: A procedure in which a surgeon examines the pelvic organs and treats for endometriosis.

Luteal Phase: Final stage of the menstrual cycle; the ruptured part of the follicle sits in the uterus until it is shed in menstruation.

Menarche: A girl's first period.

Menorrhagia: Heavy periods.

Menstruation: First stage of the menstruation cycle, where the inner lining of the uterine wall breaks down and sheds through the vagina.

Metrorrhagia: Bleeding or spotting between your normal menstruation.

Mons Pubis: Fatty area surrounding the pelvic bone that grows hair during puberty.

OB-GYN: Also spelt OB/GYN; a dual acronym for obstetrics (OB) and gynaecology (GYN). A physician who works specifically with the female reproductive system and reproductive health.

Oligomenorrhea: Irregular periods.

Ovaries: Where the woman's eggs are stored and produce hormones, connected to the fallopian tubes.

Ovulation: Third stage of the menstruation cycle; when a mature egg is released from the ovary.

Pelvic Exam: Visual and physical inspection of a woman's reproductive system. Doctors view all organs in the system to make sure everything is healthy.

Pelvic Inflammatory Disease: Inflammation of the female genital tract, accompanied by fever and lower abdominal pain.

Perimenopause: Transition toward menopause, when the ovaries start producing less estrogen.

Premenstrual Dysphoric Disorder: Condition in which a woman has severe depression symptoms, irritability, and tension before menstruation - much worse than a standard premenstrual syndrome.

Premenstrual Syndrome: Physical and emotional symptoms that occur in the one to two weeks before a woman's period.

Premenstrual Tension: Physical and emotional symptoms that occur in the one to two weeks before a woman's period.

Progesterone: Steroid hormone that readies the endometrium in case of pregnancy after the ovulation stage. Helps influence the body to ready itself to have a baby.

Polycystic Ovary Syndrome: Condition that affects a woman's hormone levels producing higher-than-normal amounts of androgens, causing them to skip menstrual periods and makes it harder for them to get pregnant.

Polyps (cervical and endometrial): Benign growths on the inside of the womb or cervix.

Progestin: Form of progesterone, this hormone functions to help prevent ovulation and stop sperm from reaching the egg by thickening the mucus in the cervix.

Septic Arthritis: Infection in a joint.

Serotonin: Hormone released during exercise that helps to improve sleep and sexual function.

Sexually Transmitted Infections: Infections that are transmitted by direct or indirect sexual contact. Can be spread through discharge, semen, or blood.

Swyer Syndrome: Condition in which the uterus and fallopian tubes (if applicable) form and function normally, but the gonads (ovaries and testes, as applicable) do not function.

Testosterone: Androgen sex hormone produced in the gonads (testes or ovaries, as applicable); it is responsible for sexual desire and aggressive characteristics.

Toxic Shock Syndrome (TSS): Rare, albeit life-threatening bacterial infection caused by toxins released by staph bacteria; in the case of menstruation, it's caused when an individual leaves a tampon in for too long (build-up of bacteria).

Trichomoniasis: Infection caused by parasitic trichomonads, commonly affecting the urinary tract, vagina, or digestive system.

Turner Syndrome: Condition in which one of a (female) person's X chromosomes is either missing or altered, usually resulting in an early loss of function in the ovaries.

Urethral Opening: Where the bladder connects to the outside of the body and where urine is expelled.

Urinalysis: A urine test.

Uterus: Where a fetus develops. The cervix also allows sperm to enter the reproductive system and menstrual blood to be expelled.

Vagina: Canal that joins the cervix, or the lower part of the uterus, it both on the inside and outside of the body.

Vaginal Discharge: Fluid and cells that are shed through the vagina that varies in colour and consistency and can indicate your vaginal health.

Vaginal Ring: Small, flexible contraceptive ring that stays in the vagina for three weeks.

Vulva: Outermost part of the female reproductive system made up of the mons pubis, clitoris, labia majora, labia minora, urethral opening, vagina, and anus.

Yeast Infections: Infection of the vagina caused by a fungus known as Candida.

FUN FACTS

Use these fun facts as ice breakers to talk to your mothers, daughters, or girlfriends about menstruation.

❖ The average woman has 400 periods during her lifetime — that totals to about four to six years of bleeding!

❖ While all mammals go through gestation and birth babies (rather than hatching them), only primates, elephants, shrews, and bats experience a monthly menstrual cycle as humans do.

❖ A woman is born with all the eggs she will ever produce. This means that when your grandmother was pregnant with your mother, she was also carrying you via your mother's eggs!

❖ Of the one to two million eggs a girl is born with, only about 500 will be released through menstruation.

❖ Most women have period stains in every pair of underwear they own, so don't feel bad. You can wear panty liners in between your periods in order to avoid stains.

❖ As recently as the 1950s, women were diagnosed with female hysteria, which was categorized by symptoms such as outbursts, irritability, sleeplessness, anxiety, increased vaginal lubrication, and sexual fantasies.

❖ On average, women go through 12,000 to 15,000 pads, tampons, and panty liners in their lifetime of menstruation.

❖ Orgasms can help reduce period pain and make your cramps feel better by letting out pain-fighting neurotransmitters such as endorphins and oxytocin.

❖ In the 1700s, the menopause was seen as a deadly disease and was treated with things like leeches to the genitalia and cervix and eclectic therapy, opium, and arsenic in the 1800s and 1900s.

❖ Women who have a higher soy diet tend to have a lower libido

❖ Some of the first tampons were small pieces of wood wrapped with lint.

❖ Ocular vicarious menstruation is a very rare period disorder that can cause bleeding in the eyes.

❖ The pill was not the first oral contraception; it was a plant called silphion, which was used in the Greek-Roman empire and was harvested to extinction.

❖ If you experience menopause before the age of forty, it is considered early menopause.

❖ Most of the people involved in developing modern birth control for women have been men.

❖ Tampons have been used in attempts to avoid unwanted pregnancy — I absolutely do not suggest this!

❖ Your period can worsen your asthma symptoms.

❖ Birth control did not become legal for everyone until 1972, the same year hacky sacks and pong were born.

❖ On average, women experience menopause at about age fifty-one.

❖ An IUD can rip the head off a sperm.

❖ The sound of your voice can change during your period.

❖ Sleeping with a night light on can help to regulate your menstrual cycle.

❖ While IUDs are very effective, we still aren't completely sure as to how they work.

❖ Your risk of heart disease can increase after you have reached menopause.

❖ Tampons are sold in packs of eighteen, as that is generally how many a woman uses during her period.

❖ The main ingredient in the birth control pill comes from yams.

❖ Modern condoms wouldn't be possible without vulcanized rubber thanks to Charles Goodyear, as in Goodyear tires.

❖ Menstrual products can soak up more than just period blood; you can keep a pad or two in your first aid kit to help with blood loss in case of another emergency.

❖ Back in the 1940s and 1950s, religious leaders thought that inserting a tampon was used for arousal.

❖ The first human trials of the birth control pill were conducted using psychiatric patients, who could not technically give their consent.

❖ In many places throughout the world, tampons and other sanitary products are still taxed as a luxury product.

❖ Before the 1970s, no one would talk about periods and menstruation in order to preserve a woman's modesty.

❖ Menstrual cups can be worn for four hours longer than tampons.

❖ In 1940, Walt Disney made a movie about periods called "The Story of Menstruation."

❖ The first tampon was patented by a man in 1931.

REFERENCES

American College of Obstetricians and Gynecologists. (2015). Dysmenorrhea: Painful periods. *The American College of Obstetricians.* Retrieved August 19, 2019, from https://www.acog.org/Patients/FAQs/Dysmenorrhea-Painful-Periods?IsMobileSet=false

American Pregnancy Association. (2019, July 9). Ovulation: Understanding ovulation cycles. *American Pregnancy Association.* Retrieved August 14, 2019, from https://americanpregnancy.org/getting-pregnant/understanding-ovulation/

BetterHealth. (2014, April 30). Menstrual cycle. *Better Health Channel.* Retrieved August 13, 2019, from https://www.betterhealth.vic.gov.au/health/conditionsandtreatments/menstrual-cycle

Bodyform. (2016, December 8). All about periods - Period myths. *Bodyform.* Retrieved August 11, 2019, from https://www.bodyform.co.uk/v-zone/your-first-period/period-myths/

Brennan, D. (2019, April 18). All about menstruation. *WebMD.* Retrieved August 13, 2019, from https://teens.webmd.com/girls/all-about-menstruation

Canadian Cancer Society. (n.d.). Hormonal therapy. *Canadian Cancer Society*. Retrieved August 31, 2019 from https://www.cancer.ca/en/cancer-information/diagnosis-and-treatment/chemotherapy-and-other-drug-therapies/hormonal-therapy/?region=on

Carter, A. (2017, September 18). Choosing between the birth control pill or the Depo-Provera shot. *Healthline*. Retrieved August 29, 2019, from https://www.healthline.com/health/birth-control/birth-control-pill-vs-shot

Castleman, M. (2015, March 15). How the menstrual cycle affects women's libido. *Psychology Today*. Retrieved from https://www.psychologytoday.com/ca/blog/all-about-sex/201503/how-the-menstrual-cycle-affects-womens-libido

Center for Young Women's Health. (2016, May 6). Period products: Information about tampons, pads, and more. *Center for Young Women's Health*. Retrieved August 29, 2019 from https://youngwomenshealth.org/2013/03/28/period-products/

Center for Young Women's Health. (2017). Sexually transmitted infections (STIs): General information. *Center for Young Women's Health*. Retrieved August 31, 2019 from https://youngwomenshealth.org/2013/01/16/sti-information/

Center for Young Women's Health. (2019, May 16). Trichomoniasis: Trichomonal vaginitis; "Trich." *Center for Young Women's Health*. Retrieved August 13, 2019 from https://youngwomenshealth.org/2012/12/11/trichomoniasis/

Clue. (2017, September 24). 36 superstitions about periods from around the world. *Clue*. Retrieved August 11, 2019, from https://helloclue.com/articles/culture/36-superstitions-about-periods-from-around-world

Cohut, M. (2019, February 8). 5 menstruation myths you must leave behind. *Medical News Today*. Retrieved from https://www.medicalnewstoday.com/articles/324403.php

Cora. (2019, August 22). The low down on the tampon tax in the US. *Cora*. Retrieved from https://cora.life/blogs/day-one/tampon-tax-in-the-us

Cornforth, T. (2019, June 26). What you should know about the endometrium. *Very Well Health*. Retrieved August 31, 2019 from https://www.verywellhealth.com/what-is-the-endometrium-2721857

Cousins, S. (2019, January 6). In Nepal, tradition is killing women. *Foreign Policy*. Retrieved from https://foreignpolicy.com/2019/01/06/in-nepal-tradition-is-killing-women-chhaupadi-womens-rights-menstruation/

Di Notto, P. M., Newman, L., Wall, S., & Einstein, G. (2013, May). The *Her*munculus: What is known about the representation of the female body in the brain? *Cerebral Cortex, 23*(5), 1005-1013. doi:10.1093/cercor/bhs005

Dowshen, S. (2015, October 1). Everything you wanted to know about puberty (for teens). *KidsHealth*. Retrieved August 13, 2019, from https://kidshealth.org/en/teens/puberty.html

Druet, A. (2017, September 7). How did menstruation become taboo? *Clue*. Retrieved from https://helloclue.com/articles/culture/how-did-menstruation-become-taboo

Drugs.com. (2019, August 9). Implanon implant: Side effects, dosage & uses. *Drugs.com*. Retrieved August 28, 2019, from https://www.drugs.com/implanon.html

Dusenbery, M. (2017, June 25). Timeline: Female hysteria and the sex toys used to treat it. *Mother Jones*. Retrieved from https://www.motherjones.com/media/2012/06/hysteria-sex-toy-history-timeline/

Ellis, D. R. (2018, July 30). Everything you need to know about vaginal discharge. *Healthline*. Retrieved August 31, 2019 from https://www.healthline.com/health/vaginal-discharge

Ellis, M. E. (2019, May 11). No menstruation (absent menstruation). *Healthline*. Retrieved August 20, 2019, from https://www.healthline.com/health/menstruation-absent

Ernst, H. (2018, August 3). Birth control patch side effects. *Healthline*. Retrieved August 29, 2019, from https://www.healthline.com/health/birth-control-patch-side-effects

Gallagher, S. (2017, April 20). 8 things everyone needs to know about having period sex. *The Huffington Post*. Retrieved from https://www.huffingtonpost.co.uk/entry/sex-on-your-period-can-you-have_uk_58f86a10e4b091e58f3861fe?guccounter=

1

Gunnars, K. (2019, January 28). Blue light and sleep: What's the connection? *Healthline*. Retrieved August 29, 2019, from https://www.healthline.com/nutrition/block-blue-light-to-sleep-better

Gupta, S. & Pokharel, S. (2019, January 11). Banished from home for menstruating, mother and two children die in Nepali hut. *CNN Health*. Retrieved from https://www.cnn.com/2019/01/10/health/menstrual-hut-death-nepal-intl/index.html

Healthwise Staff. (2018, May 15). Laparoscopic surgery for endometriosis. *HealthLink BC*. Retrieved September 5, 2019, from https://www.healthlinkbc.ca/health-topics/hw101171

Hirsch, L. (2019, June 1). Female reproductive system (for teens). *KidsHealth*. Retrieved August 13, 2019, from https://kidshealth.org/en/teens/female-repro.html

Home Health UK. (2017, October 10). Pre-menstrual syndrome (P.M.S.) and pre-menstrual tension (P.M.T.). *Home Health UK*. Retrieved August 19, 2019, from https://homehealth-uk.com/pmsandpmt/

Hormone Health Network. (n.d.). What is progesterone? *Hormone Health Network*. Retrieved from https://www.hormone.org/your-health-and-hormones/glands-and-hormones-a-to-z/hormones/progesterone

Johnson, T. C. (2018, December 12). Your guide to the female reproductive system. *WebMD*. Retrieved August 11, 2019, from https://www.webmd.com/sex-relationships/guide/your-guide-female-reproductive-system

Kane, S. (2018, July 5). 10 surprising health benefits of mindfulness meditation. *Psych Central*. Retrieved from https://psychcentral.com/blog/10-surprising-health-benefits-of-mindfulness-meditation/

Kennedy, S., Bergqvist, A., Chapron, C., D'Hooghe, T., Dunselman, G., Greb, R., Saridogan, E. (2005, June 24). ESHRE guideline for the diagnosis and treatment of endometriosis. *Human Reproduction, 20*(10), 2698-2704. doi:10.1093/humrep/dei135

Klepchukova, A. (2018, December 7). Exercising during period: Benefits and things to avoid. *Flo*. Retrieved from https://flo.health/menstrual-cycle/lifestyle/fitness-and-exercise/exercising-during-period

Lama, S. C. (2018, December 18). Why do I crave sweets during my period? *Livestrong.com*. Retrieved August 31, 2019 from https://www.livestrong.com/article/460961-why-do-i-crave-sweets-during-my-period/

Liu, Y., Gold, E. B., Lasley, B. L., & Johnson, W. O. (2004). Factors affecting menstrual cycle characteristics. *American Journal of Epidemiology*, *160*(2), 131–140. doi:10.1093/aje/kwh188

MacLeod, N. (2018). Libido and your menstrual cycle. *Menstruation.com*. Retrieved August 20, 2019, from https://www.menstruation.com.au/periodpages/libido.html

Mayo Clinic Staff. (2017, May 7). Perimenopause: Symptoms and causes. *Mayo Clinic*. Retrieved August 20, 2019, from https://www.mayoclinic.org/diseases-conditions/perimenopause/symptoms-causes/syc-20354666

Mayo Clinic Staff. (2017, May 25). Birth control pill FAQ: Benefits, risks and choices. *Mayo Clinic*. Retrieved August 21, 2019, from https://www.mayoclinic.org/healthy-lifestyle/birth-control/in-depth/birth-control-pill/art-20045136

Mayo Clinic Staff. (2018, May 4). Trichomoniasis: Diagnosis and treatment. *Mayo Clinic.* Retrieved August 14, 2019, from https://www.mayoclinic.org/diseases-conditions/trichomoniasis/diagnosis-treatment/drc-20378613

Mayo Clinic Staff. (2019, May 1). Bacterial vaginosis. *Mayo Clinic.* Retrieved August 14, 2019, from https://www.mayoclinic.org/diseases-conditions/bacterial-vaginosis/symptoms-causes/syc-20352279

Mayo Clinic Staff. (2019, July 16). Yeast infection (vaginal): Diagnosis and treatment - *Mayo Clinic.* Retrieved August 14, 2019, from https://www.mayoclinic.org/diseases-conditions/yeast-infection/diagnosis-treatment/drc-20379004

Mayo Clinic Staff. (2019, July 25). Gonorrhea. *Mayo Clinic.* Retrieved August 14, 2019, from https://www.mayoclinic.org/diseases-conditions/gonorrhea/symptoms-causes/syc-20351774

Meyer, R., & Fetters, A. (2018, September 6). Victorian-era orgasms and the crisis of peer review. *The Atlantic.* Retrieved from https://www.theatlantic.com/health/archive/2018/09/victorian-vibrators-orgasms-doctors/569446/

Miller, J. (2019, August 11). Top 10 period myths busted. *Kotex*. Retrieved from https://www.ubykotex.com/en-us/periods/period-advice/top-10-period-myths-busted

National Health Service Direct Wales. (2019, May 22). Menorrhagia. *NHS Direct Wales*. Retrieved August 19, 2019, from https://www.nhsdirect.wales.nhs.uk/encyclopaedia/m/article/menorrhagia/

National Health Service. (2018, December 10). PMS (premenstrual syndrome). *NHS*. Retrieved August 19, 2019, from https://www.nhs.uk/conditions/pre-menstrual-syndrome/

National Health Service. (2019, August 12). Delayed periods. *NHS*. Retrieved August 13, 2019, from https://www.nhs.uk/conditions/periods/delayed-periods/

Nichols, H. (2018, January 2). Everything you need to know about estrogen. *Medical News Today*. Retrieved August 31, 2019 from https://www.medicalnewstoday.com/articles/277177.php

OBOS Anatomy & Menstruation Contributors. (2014, 1 April). Stages in the menstrual cycle. *Our Bodies Ourselves*. Retrieved August 30, 2019, from https://www.ourbodiesourselves.org/book-excerpts/health-article/stages-in-the-menstrual-cycle/

Pandia Health. (2019, June 20). Bleeding while using birth control: What's normal? *Pandia Health*. Retrieved August 24, 2019, from https://www.pandiahealth.com/birth-control/bleeding

Piedmont Healthcare. (2019, August 11). How exercise helps balance hormones. *Piedmont Healthcare*. Retrieved August 11, 2019, from https://www.piedmont.org/living-better/how-exercise-helps-balance-hormones

Pietrangelo, A., & Cherney, K. (2018, December 21). The effects of hormonal birth control on your body. *Healthline*. Retrieved August 21, 2019, from https://www.healthline.com/health/birth-control-effects-on-body

Planned Parenthood. (2019). What is premenstrual dysphoric disorder? *Planned Parenthood*. Retrieved August 19, 2019, from https://www.plannedparenthood.org/learn/health-and-wellness/menstruation/what-premenstrual-dysphoric-disorder-pmdd

Rowland, A. S., Baird, D. D., Long, S., Wegienka, Harlow, S. D., Alavanja, M., & Sandler, D. P. (2002, November). Influence of medical conditions and lifestyle factors on the menstrual cycle. *Epidemiology, 13*(6), 668-674. doi:10.1097/01.EDE.0000024628.42288.8F

Santos-Longhurst, A. (2018, August 1). 14 possible causes for irregular periods. *Medical News Today*. Retrieved from https://www.medicalnewstoday.com/articles/3226 43.php

Seladi-Schulman, J. (2019, March 1). Everything you need to know about chlamydia infection. *Healthline*. Retrieved August 14, 2019, from https://www.healthline.com/health/std/chlamydia

Sigurðardóttir, E. R. (2013, September). Women and madness in the 19th century: The effects of oppression on women's mental health. *Háskóli Íslands Hugvísindasvið*. Retrieved from https://skemman.is/bitstream/1946/16449/1/BA -ElisabetRakelSigurdar.pdf

Sharma, J. (2019, March 13). The state of period poverty in the United States. *Paper Magazine*. Retrieved August 22, 2019, from https://www.papermag.com/period-poverty- tampon-tax-united-states-2631311601.html

Shkodzik, K. (2019, June 1). What happens after stopping birth control? Weight gain, bleeding, and other symptoms. *Flo*. Retrieved from https://flo.health/menstrual-cycle/sex/birth-control/what-happens-after-stopping-birth-control

Sissons, C. (2018, May 15). What causes bleeding between periods? *Medical News Today*. Retrieved August 20, 2019, from https://www.medicalnewstoday.com/articles/321811.php

Stöppler, M. C. (2019, March 26). 25 ways to relieve menstrual cramps. Retrieved August 22, 2019, from https://www.onhealth.com/content/1/menstrual_period_cramps

Sullivan, D. (2018, September 18). What is breakthrough bleeding and why does it happen? *Healthline*. Retrieved August 23, 2019, from https://www.healthline.com/health/womens-health/breakthrough-bleeding

Tampax. (2019). How to feel better on your period. *Tampax*. Retrieved from https://tampax.com/en-us/tips-and-advice/period-advice/how-to-feel-better-on-your-period

Tanner, C. (Writer), & Briganti, P. (Director). (2015, December 8). Adam ruins sex [Adam ruins everything episode]. In P. Briganti (Producer),

Adam ruins everything. Hollywood, CA: Big Breakfast.

Tantry, T. (2019, January 4). Spotting on birth control: When to start worrying about it? *Flo.* Retrieved from https://flo.health/menstrual-cycle/sex/birth-control/spotting-on-birth-control

Todd, N. (2019, April 2). Understanding toxic shock syndrome -- The basics. *WebMD.* Retrieved August 21, 2019, from https://www.webmd.com/women/guide/understanding-toxic-shock-syndrome-basics

Traniello, V. (n.d.). Hysteria and the wandering womb. *Marquette University.* Retrieved from https://academic.mu.edu/meissnerd/hysteria.html#Web

Vergnaud, S. (2019, February 6). Can my medications interfere with my birth control? *GoodRX.* Retrieved from https://www.goodrx.com/blog/can-medications-make-birth-control-less-effective/

Werft, M., & Canal, G. (2017, May 23). Ten myths about periods. *Global Citizen.* Retrieved from https://www.globalcitizen.org/en/content/8-crazy-cultural-myths-about-periods/

Wischhover, C. (2019, July 10). Breaking the hymen: 6 facts and myths about virginity. *Teen Vogue.* Retrieved from https://www.teenvogue.com/story/facts-about-hymen-and-virginity

WomenLog. (2019). Travel & your period. *WomenLog.* Retrieved August 22, 2019, from https://www.womanlog.com/cycle/travel-your-period

www.ingramcontent.com/pod-product-compliance
Lightning Source LLC
Chambersburg PA
CBHW031100250726

48655CB00004B/1518